Who Can Ride the Dragon?

Who Can Ride the *Dragon?*

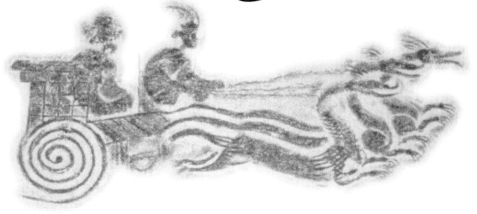

An Exploration of the Cultural Roots of
Traditional Chinese Medicine

ZHANG YU HUAN

and KEN ROSE

PARADIGM PUBLICATIONS

Who Can Ride the Dragon?
An Exploration of the Cultural Roots of Traditional Chinese Medicine

Copyright © 1995, 1996, 1997, 1998, 1999
by Zhang Yu Huan and Ken Rose
ISBN # 0-912111-59-3

Library of Congress Cataloging-In-Publication Information:
Zhang Yu Huan, 1973-
    Who can ride the dragon? : an exploration of the cultural roots
of traditional Chinese medicine / by Zhang Yu Huan and Ken Rose.
    p. cm.
Includes bibliographical references (p. 257) and index.
ISBN 0-91-211159-3 (alk. paper)
1. Medicine, Chinese. I. Rose, Ken, 1952- II. Title.
R601 .H758 1999
610'.951--dc21
                    99-6702
                    CIP

Printed in the United States of America

PARADIGM PUBLICATIONS
http://www.paradigm-pubs.com
44 Linden Street, Brookline, Massachusetts 02445 USA
Publisher: Robert L. Felt
Cover Design by Laura Shaw Design

for David Wakefield
1950~1999
In Memoriam

Contents

DESIGNATION

Paradigm Publications is a participant in the Council of Oriental Medical Publishers (C.O.M.P.) and supports their effort to make readers aware of the sources of East Asian medical information and the methods used to represent it in English. By C.O.M.P. guidelines, this work is an "original work."

Unless otherwise noted or quoted, the authors follow the translational nomenclature from Wiseman and Feng, *A Practical Dictionary of Chinese Medicine,* Paradigm Publications, Brookline, MA, 1998.

About the Cover Illustration and Calligraphy

The dragon image used on the cover and throughout the text derives from a rubbing taken from a Han Dynasty tomb discovered in the 1980's in Peng Xian township outside Chengdu, the capital of Sichuan Province in southwest China. The dragon chariot portrayed is a symbol of the magical power the ancients wished to preserve for their descendants. 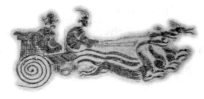 Here, three dragons draw the two primary aspects of consciousness. The wheel of the chariot is an ancient symbol of eternity.

The calligraphy throughout the text was executed by Peng Shi Qing of Chengdu, China. We extend our gratitude to him for sharing the bounty of his art.

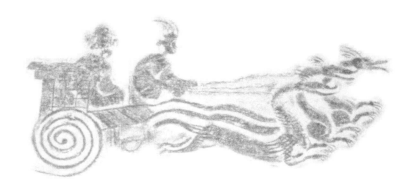

ACKNOWLEDGEMENTS

A book such as this gives expression to ideas that have been developing for a very long time. Although we assume ultimate responsibility for the contents, we wish to acknowledge the participation of many people whose time, attention, effort, teaching, research, and support make our own work possible.

We want to thank the faculty, staff, and student body of the Chengdu University of Traditional Chinese Medicine for their spirited cooperation over the years. President Li Ming Fu has been especially supportive of our efforts, and Prof. Huang Qing Xian has worked hard to provide a practical basis for ongoing cooperation. Wang Zhi Fu, Director of the Library, generously made it possible for us to have access to the antiquarian book collection there. A special thanks goes to the students who took part in the graduate seminar on the translation of Chinese medical terms and texts.

Without the love and support of our families, we would be lost. We owe a special debt of gratitude to Zhang Guang Tai and Guo Long Hui for putting up with us through freezing winters and melting summer heat. To Aaron and Balyn, who put up with more than is reasonable, we can only say, "Thank you."

We are particularly indebted to our editors, Bob Felt and Martha Fielding, for the painstaking work they have done on our manuscript. Without their steady hands guiding the process, this book may not have come into being. "Good books take time," they said at the outset. And if this book achieves a measure of goodness, it is proof of that assertion and of the quality of their work. Thanks to Rod Sperry for laboring with the book inside and out, and to the crew at Paradigm for all their hard work.

Special thanks also go to Irene Speiser who read the manuscript at an early stage and helped to knock some of the rough edges off. Irene's love and support have kept us moving forward.

As we find ourselves at the beginning of a new millenium, we must admit to having a particularly poignant awareness of our debt to the muted voices of the past, the countless doctors and patients whose relentless search for health has resulted in a culture of wellbeing that we believe has much to offer the modern world.

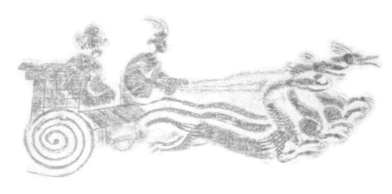

FOREWORD

by Harriet Beinfield, co-author with Efrem Korngold,
Between Heaven and Earth: A Guide to Chinese Medicine

THE ESSAYIST ANATOLE BROYARD, in the midst of struggling with prostate cancer, wrote in his journal, "Illness is a kind of incoherence." Medicine is an attempt to remedy incoherence by generating systematic explanatory models from which healing techniques are devised.

Medical ideas are neither free-floating nor arbitrary—they do not sail through space like particles of dust caught by the wind. They arise from traditions of thought and habits of mind deeply embedded within a social context. Chinese medicine is sometimes misconstrued as being singularly synonomous with its instrumental techniques, particularly acupuncture and herbal medicine. Rather, it is less confined, expressing modes of knowing (epistemology), beliefs about the nature of reality (metaphysics), and theories of human experience (physiology, psychology, theology), as well as positing methods of being helpful (therapeutic interventions). Because every medicine is situated at the intersection of biological and cultural highways, it is valuable to grasp the cultural coding that shapes it. How is its meaning generated? From whence does it arise? How has Chinese medical thought been socially constructed to form the complex matrix that constitutes its explanatory model?

Chinese medicine has spread like a slow-burning grass fire across America's cultural fields. It is appreciated for its practical value: people ailing are made to feel better. It has seduced many thousands of students to spend countless hours in dedicated study. Part of its appeal is in its exotic wisdom that reaches several millenia back through time, distillations of which have filtered through history to reach us now, on our distant shore. Still, the mountains of knowledge within the terrain of Chinese medicine are not altogether accessible to the ordinary Western mind. While its mystery is tolerated, that parts of it remain mystified and bewildering is a source of consternation.

Many of the schools of Chinese medicine in the West have concentrated on the pragmatic task of producing practitioners, attentive to enabling students to acquire the education and the skills required for licensure and practice. The daunting task of assuming responsibility for the transmission of cultural knowledge is often neglected. Anthropologists are familiar with the phenomenon of inhabitants of a given clime mistaking the quirks of their idiosyncratic world as simply "the way things are." Teasing out these taken-for-granted assumptions, patterns, and conventions is their metier. Still, historian Robert Darnton comments, "One thing seems clear to everyone who returns from field work: other people are other. They do not think the way we do."

Who Can Ride the Dragon? provides a cultural translation of a foreign conceptual language. The authors decode linguistic differences between English and Chinese, describe ancient beliefs and customs, expose philosophical roots, literary and scientific traditions, develop an historical overview of Chinese medical and sexual culture, and explain key terms. The authors each speak an adopted language: Ken Rose travels from the West toward the East, while Zhang Yu Huan journeys from the East toward the West. Together, they have performed a great service by clearing a path into the formidably dense thicket that constitutes Chinese medicine in the West. This text provides a select and decipherable site map, a window of inestimable value into a world of meaning that satisfies a yearning on the part of many who hunger to know the substrate from which Chinese medicine emerges.

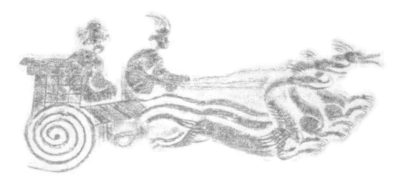

OUR ARGUMENT IS SIMPLE.

Chinese medicine is a cultural phenomenon. To understand it and to use it properly you must first acquire a thorough familiarity with its cultural background. Only thus can its deeper meanings be fully assimilated and appreciated.

Without investigating and considering its cultural substrate, the theories and methods of Chinese medicine lose their multidimensionality and become quaint—even bizarre—artifacts. In the hands of those who lack such understanding, the medical methods and substances do not function effectively.

Interest in Chinese medicine has dramatically increased in the past several decades. Schools of acupuncture have sprung up around the world. Yet, for the most part, the curriculum in these schools stresses technical and mechanical considerations, leaving the cultural matrix, the living root of Chinese traditional medicine, under- or unrepresented.

This is understandable for many reasons. China has only recently reopened its doors to foreigners to provide, for the first time in a half-century, greater access to the archives and, more importantly, the living experience of traditional Chinese culture. To be sure, Chinese culture has experienced a lengthy diaspora resulting in overseas Chinese communities around the world. In these enclaves Chinese traditional medicine has been steadily practiced but, for the most part, confined to Chinese and other Asians for whom the cultural aspects of Chinese medicine pose fewer problems.

There have been many notable forays into the mind/heart of traditional Chinese culture. Yet in comparison to a vast cultural development of ten thousand years, we have only begun to scratch the surface of subjects such as Chinese medicine. The aim of this book is thus several fold.

First, we want to draw attention to the magnitude of the study implied by the cultural aspects of the traditional medicine of China. We have attempted to do this as one might define a circle or sphere, not by drawing every peripheral point but by concentrating on the central issues, on the essence of the subject.

Second, we wish to create inroads, regardless of how difficult and narrow they may be, into the density of this cultural substrate.

Third, we hope to provide some assistance to those students, doctors, patients, and others who seek a richer and deeper understanding of Chinese medicine.

Finally, we want to provide an enjoyable reading experience, to move your mind and your imagination with the words of the story we tell.

To the degree that we succeed in these, our aim is achieved. We have begun our work with the full awareness that we cannot complete it. It is the beauty and wonder of the subject itself that has sustained us through the years of our endeavor.

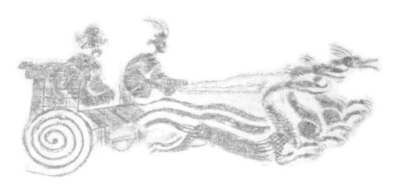

A Note Regarding Pīnyīn and Tones

THROUGHOUT THIS BOOK we have employed the standard method in use in mainland China today of writing Chinese words with Roman letters. This system is known as Pīnyīn. Pīnyīn literally means "spell sound." It was adopted as part of an overall plan to deal with the wide varieties of regional speech so that the whole country could enjoy the benefits of a single language standard. Despite the efforts of scholars and officials to develop a widely used Romanized version of Chinese, this system is not widely relied upon in daily life in China where people still use the written characters for writing and reading their language. The method we have employed follows the 1956 standardization, which is used throughout China as part of this overall effort to standardize the language throughout the country.

One of the purposes of these efforts to standardize the writing of Chinese in Roman letters is to make the language more accessible to foreigners. Yet even this raises as many questions as it answers. A Chinese teacher once advised against the use of Pīnyīn, pointing out that it simply gave the poor, frustrated foreigner struggling valiantly to learn Chinese yet one more set of symbols to have to contend with.

Perhaps he also had the poor authors and publishers of books in English that deal with Chinese language in mind. Here is what we have done. In order to make the book as readable as possible, yet still provide readers with access to the Chinese sounds of the words, we have used toned Pīnyīn for all Chinese words with the exception of people's names and place names. We decided to exclude these names as a method of identifying the names of people and places more easily in the text. Whenever a Chinese word appears in the text that does not have a tone mark above it, it is the name of a place or a person.

What is toned Pīnyīn? In standard Chinese there are four tones employed in the pronunciation of words. The first tone or high tone, neither falling nor rising, is noted as "‾". The second tone, which rises from the beginning to the end of the word, is noted as " ´ ". The third tone, which falls and then rises, is noted as " ˇ " . The fourth tone, which falls from beginning to end, is noted as "ˋ". There is a fifth or neutral (unstressed) tone in standard Chinese. When a word is spoken in the neutral (fifth) tone, it is written without any tone mark in Pīnyīn.

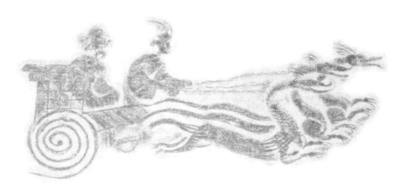

INTRODUCTION

THIS BOOK IS INTENDED to aid the study of Chinese traditional medicine. It is for students, doctors, teachers, researchers, patients, healthcare professionals, and anyone else who needs insight into the cultural background of Chinese traditional medicine.

We have made several assumptions: First, we assume that individuals born and raised outside of China and the cultural context of the Chinese language have no background from which to draw when faced with the subtle and complex difficulties of understanding Chinese traditional medicine. Some of these may seem vast and overwhelming, while others are so subtle as to go unnoticed. The list of chapter and section headings in the table of contents are the difficulties that we have chosen to address. Second, we assume that readers will use this book in conjunction with other fine materials already available. Likewise, we assume that readers will avail themselves of new materials as these become available. Although it has been steadily undertaken for several decades now, the translation and publication of Chinese traditional medical materials in English and other Western languages has really just begun. Third, we assume that we will be taken as gatherers and presenters rather than as "authorities" on Chinese medicine. It is not our intention to create or establish definitive or authoritative interpretations. We simply wish to engage in the exposition of insights into this vast and complex subject. In this respect, we welcome and invite readers' criticisms, comments, and suggestions for improvement.

Chinese medicine is truly a cultural phenomenon. Its continued development depends on the fundamental processes of culture. Among these, none is more basic nor more important than the use of language to communicate, exchange, and refine ideas. Thus our text begins with a discussion of the Chinese language and the challenges facing those who wish to understand a subject that originates in the traditions, beliefs, and written records of the Chinese people.

This book is not a textbook. Nor is it a dictionary. Instead, you will find in it broad discussions of the language of Chinese traditional medicine—terms, words, phrases, and ideas that, taken together, form the matrix from which the subject has evolved.

There may seem to be a "chicken or egg" dilemma facing those who would untangle the knot of complicated interrelationships that exists between medical theories and practices and the cultural roots that underlie and support them. The approach we have taken reflects our own needs, strengths, and weaknesses as we have worked to resolve these difficulties for ourselves. It takes a lifetime to master even the sub-disciplines of Chinese medicine. Our work is only a beginning.

With all this in mind, the sections of this book should not be considered as the categorical imperatives of the subject. Rather, they emerged as convenient subdivisions that allowed us to sort and sift this complex material as we established our own foundation of understanding.

WHO CAN RIDE THE DRAGON?

Our search to discover the roots of traditional medicine in China continues to lead us into breathtaking territories that we once only imagined. Indeed, the charm and allure of Chinese medicine is composed of many aspects and ingredients. While sorting, compiling, and making sense of the thousands of pages of research—clinical and miscellaneous notes we have collected through the years of our study—some very clear questions have emerged. At its heart, Chinese medicine contains a substantial portion of what Lao Zi called "mystery upon mystery." Delving into mysteries can be rewarding but it has its requirements.

The Chinese people have long considered themselves to be "children of the dragon." But what precisely is the dragon? The dragon is a beast that embodies mysteries. Whether ruling a kingdom deep beneath the sea or soaring beyond the clouds to deliver a message to the lord of the Ninth Heaven, the dragon moves through Chinese mythology with fierce power. It is a symbol for everything Chinese. Here we evoke its image only to frame our indelicate question: Who can ride the dragon?

In his preface to the long-revered and intensely studied classic, *Prescriptions Worth a Thousand Pieces of Gold*, the Tang Dynasty physician Sun Si Miao stated the following on preparing to study the art of healing:

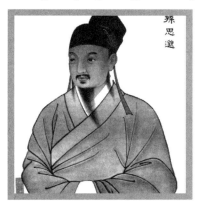

Prerequisites for the Study of Medicine:
Whoever wants to be a doctor must first be conversant with Sù Wèn, Jiá Yí, Huáng Dì Zhēn Jīn, the twelve channels, the three places and nine depths [for taking the pulse], the five zàng and six fú organs, the exterior and the interior, the points that lie along the channels, medicinals, and all other well-known books of doctors and formulas such as Zhang Zhong Jing [Shāng Hán Lùn], Wang Su He, Ruan He Nan, Fan Dong Yang, Zhang Miao, Jin Shao.

They must also understand yīn and yáng and be able to discern life's fortunes [read people's faces and see their fates]. They must also understand the cracks in the tortoise shells of Zhōu Yì [the ancient method of divination associated with the Yì Jīng and similar oracular traditions]. They must have an intimate knowledge of all these things to become a good doctor. Without such knowledge they will be like a blind person in the dark; they will fall down easily.

The next requirement is to become familiar with this book [Qiān Jīn Fāng]. Study it carefully and give it some thought. Then you can say you are on the trail of medicine. You must also engage in other reading. Why? If you do not read the Five Classics you will not understand justice, humanity, and virtue. If you do not read the Three Histories you will not know the past and the present. If you do not read the exponents of the various schools of thought, you will not understand what is happening in front of your very eyes! If you do not read the Nèi Jīng you will not know the virtue of mercy, sorrow, happiness, giving. If you do not read Zhuang Zi and Lao Zi, you will not know how to conduct your daily life.

As for the theory of the five phases, geography, astronomy . . . you also need to study these. If you can study and understand such knowledge, there is no hindrance on the road of medicine. You can become perfect.

Such advice is no less applicable today than when it was written by one of China's leading medical experts more than 1300 years ago. Indeed, we of the contemporary age are well-advised to attend to his wise suggestions. If you take these words not as a quaint historical relic but as profound wisdom meant to guide the education of medical students and professionals, you will see that like most sage advice, it is easier said than done.

China is remote from life in the West. If this is true of contemporary China, how much greater is our distance from the traditions of China's ancient past! Keep in mind that the words of Sun Si Miao were intended for Chinese students. These students already understood the Chinese language and the milieu of cultural values, precepts, and beliefs that form the substrate of the knowledge to which the great physician refered. The task for Western students is all the more difficult, for we must first be able to understand something of the way the Chinese think, feel, and express themselves to benefit from studying such materials. In our own experience, this is no easy task; it is like riding a dragon.

Thus we reiterate our simple question: Who can ride the dragon? We cannot answer the question, only ask it. We ask it not to evaluate those who would ride this marvelous creature, but rather to encourage our fellow students. It is a worthwhile challenge to demand of ourselves only the highest standard. We also hope that in the pages to follow we will provide those of you who wish to ride this dragon some measure of support and insight to assist your quest. Will we succeed? Like those who have gone before us, we can only wait and see.

CHAPTER ONE

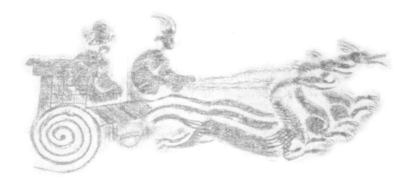

The Language of Chinese Medicine

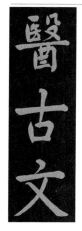

Those who know do not speak. Those who speak do not know.
—DAO DE JING

To use words wrongly is not only a fault itself; it also corrupts the soul.
—SOCRATES

THE LANGUAGE OF CHINESE MEDICINE has been developing for two thousand years. It is at once rich, complicated, and difficult to understand. Though many, if not most, contemporary Chinese consider it almost unapproachably difficult, nearly everyone in China is familiar with its basic vocabulary, for Chinese medical words are common to much of traditional Chinese culture. Naturally, this vocabulary also contains numerous technical terms. However, unlike the terminology of Western medicine, the language of Chinese medicine is derived from words that the Chinese use in their daily lives.

This fact is important to understand the language of Chinese medicine and to develop a method for comprehending the complex meanings of its words and ideas. The foundation of any such method is familiarity. Because this is not a textbook of Chinese, we are not advancing one translational method or another. Rather, we have selected examples of words and their basic characteristics that provide a foundation of familiarity. From this foundation you may choose your own course of further study. Our approach is in keeping with the values of traditional Chinese medicine and of traditional Chinese culture in general. Ultimately, it is your own intelligence, intention, and dedication that determine how well you understand the words, theories, and techniques. Chinese scholars have long recognized and respected such truth. In the two-thousand-year span of extant Chinese medical writings, they have developed a body of literature that is both a vast treasurehouse of wisdom and a considerable barrier.

A doorway exists, the language itself. It is here we begin; it is here we seek entrance.

 # THE HISTORICAL CONTEXT

Scholars of Chinese language can attest that there have been many attempts to produce standard language lexicons both in Chinese and in translation. Still, Chinese presents students with considerable barriers. It appears all the more impenetrable for those who, coming from cultures other than China, lack familiarity with the cultural basis from which the concepts and terminology of Chinese medicine arise.

Chinese medical history spans more than two millenia. Taking into account developments before written history, the span of time that concerns Chinese medical historians stretches toward 5000 years. Historical development has codified the terminology of Chinese medicine. The nomenclature has taken on a standard traditional structure over time. It is usually presented according to the main subdivisions of the subject itself. Thus comprehensive dictionaries of Chinese medicine are organized by categories such as basic theories (yīn-yáng and the five phases); the structure and function of the body organs (zàng fǔ); the material basis of vital activities (qì, blood, essence, spirit, and body fluids); etiology and pathogenesis; methods of diagnosis; and differentiation of patterns. Without a basis of study and understanding, even this arrangement can appear mysterious to those approaching Chinese medicine for the first time. Though at first glance it may seem an old and rickety structure, it remains curiously vital after thousands of years.

語 THE NATURE OF THE NOMENCLATURE

Such curious and unfamiliar arrangements can create complex and at times hidden problems for the dedicated novice studying Chinese medicine. For example, much of the terminology of Chinese medicine comes directly from ancient sources. Ancient Chinese used terse verbal structures, at once vague and profoundly meaningful. Ancient writers condensed a great deal of information into single words and brief phrases. As much as being vessels of data, knowledge, and communication, these ancient formulations are mnemonic devices meant not simply to contain and convey information, but also to connote an entire framework of knowledge. One Chinese word may be worth a lifetime's study, and then some.

At other times, the ancient language is exquisitely expressive, penetrating deeply into the poetic. The problems encountered in the study of Chinese medical terms and texts reflect the richness, depth, and profundity of the material, as well as the dense cultural fiber that supports and nourishes it. As mentioned earlier, many, probably most, contemporary Chinese avoid the undertaking. Yet in their daily life they use expressions that derive from the same source, the wellsprings of traditional Chinese wisdom.

Among the most fundamental problems faced by non-Chinese students of Chinese medicine is that many of the terms of Chinese medicine have several meanings. Even more problematic is that ancient Chinese words tend to mean all of their meanings simultaneously. The well-educated Chinese reader of ancient texts understands these various meanings in a way that is similar to the phenomenon of harmonics in acoustics: the various meanings tend to harmonize and to form an expanded sense in the mind of the reader. While this can be seen as an admirable linguistic feature, it makes translating these harmonies into familiar words in other languages an extremely difficult task. Overtones and resonances are lost. The complete meaning vanishes, leaving only a bare outline of the original composite structure.

This being the case, it is tempting to abandon the challenges of translation and simply devote our time to learning Chinese. In fact, there is no substitute for learning Chinese if you wish to explore the depths of traditional medicine and related cultural subjects. Yet, for many reasons, not the least of which is the sheer difficulty of the undertaking, most non-Chinese do not.

 ## THE BASICS OF CHINESE LANGUAGE

For those unfamiliar with Chinese it appears to be an intricate, impenetrably difficult maze of symbols and meanings. In the past, Westerners studying Chinese language, medicine, and culture in general tended to understand it in terms of their own experience. This is a natural tendency, though limited and limiting.

In approaching Chinese from English as a native language we must first recognize the difference between these two very different manifestations of the same fundamental human needs. Although it is certainly correct to call both English and Chinese "languages," the differences are many and basic. To be sure, there are numerous similarities between the two systems for conceiving, encapsulating, and transmitting meaning and messages between people. But in several important regards, each language accomplishes these ends in disparate modes and with different methods.

With respect to written English and Chinese, the symbolization of perception and thought develops in two quite different modes. English is a system of recording symbols that represent sounds. Groups of sounds are references to meaning, largely by arbitrary convention. It could be termed "sonographic" in the sense that it is a notation of speech. Even when reading silently, without articulating the sounds of the words, we recognize these sound associations. The meaning of an English sentence develops and unfolds in much the same way as a line of music. It is temporal and linear in form.

Chinese written language, on the other hand, begins in abstract pictures of thoughts/things/actions. Chinese characters and words tend to stress the relationship between things, and the abstract symbols that comprise the Chinese "alphabet" demonstrate those relationships. The meanings of Chinese words, sentences, and phrases develop from an ordering of pictographic and ideographic elements. This method, quite different from that of English, is essentially pictorial. It is spatial and spherical in form. It is a visual language that develops more like painting than music, although the music of the language is nonetheless vivid.

Written Chinese seems paradoxical in that it possesses concise formulations of meaning that are often vague references to alternate meanings. In this sense, Chinese is inclusive, that is, one Chinese word tends to include variant meanings which, as often as not, are all considered valid by those who use them. This is made clear to the beginning student of Chinese who asks, groping for understanding, "Does word 'x' mean 'a,' 'b,' or 'c'?" "Yes," answers the teacher confidently. And so it goes.

Even when words have several meanings in English, we tend to use these meanings one at a time. In contrast, Chinese tends to weave together all the various strands of connotation simultaneously to produce a thick, rich brocade of meaning. Unraveling such interwoven threads can be difficult, even impossible. The overall meaning of a Chinese expression, whether a single word or a lengthy treatise, is often a function of the multiple facets and variegated surfaces of these complex verbal structures. It is abstract pictures of ideas in dynamic interrelationship.

Let us examine an example of such a phenomenon. The Chinese character *ān* is composed of two parts. The top part, as in the character *zì*, has the meaning of a roof or covering. The bottom part is the radical. This radical, *nǔ*, also stands alone as a word meaning woman. The character, *ān*, therefore depicts a relationship between the roof of a house and a woman within. The word *ān* means "peace" or "peaceful." It is used to form other expressions such as *ān quán*, which means "safety." The character *quán* means "completely." The logic of such formulations is simple: a house with a woman inside connotes a state of peace and wellbeing. Something that is completely peaceful is, indeed, safe. The sociological implications are fascinating.

ān

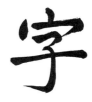

zì

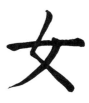

nǔ

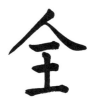

quán

The Language of Chinese Medicine

比 THE STRUCTURAL ORGANIZATION OF CHINESE COMPARED TO ENGLISH

Linguists traditionally believe that if something can be expressed in one language or one dialect it can be expressed in any other language or dialect. However, the reality of translating Chinese medical texts challenges this assumption. No translation problem more clearly exemplifies this than the difficulties that arise in defining the concept of *qì*—difficulties that require a detailed understanding. However, fundamental details of the basic structure and organization of the two languages does yield a useful comparison.

The following table compares the structural organization of the two written languages. You can see at a glance that Chinese contains a larger number of what we have called "structural elements." It is also significant that Chinese contains many more words that express aspects of the idea we term a "word" in English. Many Chinese "words" could all be translated by the English "word": *cí, zì, yán, yǔ,* and *wén.* There are many inferences that can be made from this fact. One seems most obvious: Chinese is much more self-reflexive and self-referential than English. This can be understood by analogy. For example, in the languages of peoples who live in the arctic where snow is abundant much of the year, there are far more words that mean "snow" than in the languages of people who live in the snowless tropics.

A COMPARISON OF THE STRUCTURAL ORGANIZATION OF CHINESE AND ENGLISH	
Chinese Language	
Strokes (*bǐ huà*)	6 basic strokes used to write all words
Radicals (*piān páng*)	200+ radicals
Characters (*zì*)	10,000's of characters; one must know at least several 1,000's
Words (*cí*)	100,000's of words
Idioms (*chéng yǔ*)	100,000's of idioms
English Language	
Letters	26 letters
Words	100,000's of words

Traditionally for the Chinese people, language skills—the ability to conceive, transmit, receive, and understand meaning and knowledge with words—have always been enormously important parts of cultural and intellectual life. This is variously reflected in cultural phenomena from the omnipresent wordplay of vernacular Chinese to the arcane structures of classical poetry. Clearly, the path to understanding the language of Chinese thought as it developed over thousands of years begins with an examination of the characters, the written symbols of the language.

漢字 WHAT IS A "CHARACTER" IN CHINESE?

Like so many questions about the Chinese language, this one can be answered in different ways. A Chinese character is roughly comparable to a written word in English. However, most Chinese words are composed of two characters. To distinguish between these two classes of verbal expressions—between characters and words—there are two different terms in Chinese. The character $z\grave{i}$ refers to single characters, whether or not they stand alone and function by themselves as words. The character $c\acute{i}$ refers to words that are usually two or more characters. (Refer to the table above, p. 10.)

As indicated in the table above, single characters, $z\grave{i}$, are composed of radicals. These radicals are made up of various strokes. There are many different strokes used in writing Chinese characters, but six are most commonly used. For example, the character $z\grave{i}$ is composed of two radicals. The upper part is a radical with the general meaning of "roof" or "covering." The lower part is a radical that means "son," "seed," and a variety of other things that fit a loose category of "created things."

Frequently, as in this example, it is not possible to deduce the meaning of a Chinese character by simply assembling the meanings of its parts. Nonetheless, there is an implicit developmental logic at work in the formation of Chinese characters. Although this becomes clearer only after years of study, a general impression of Chinese characters can give students of Chinese medicine a grasp of how its literature is composed.

A Chinese character can be understood as the basic functional unit of meaning in the language. Meaning is encapsulated in characters in several ways. In essence,

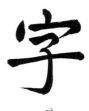

zì

upper part of zì

lower part of zì

characters evolved from an ancient picture-writing system that featured depictions of objects, actions, and considerations of the relationships that exist between them. Characters were thus associated with both meanings and sounds.

In different parts of China, different dialects are spoken. Yet all the dialects refer to the same written characters. Thus one character may have different pronunciations in different dialects. People from different parts of China may not always be able to freely converse with one another, but they all share a common written language. This has had a powerful uniting influence on the Chinese people throughout the millennia of Chinese cultural and intellectual development.

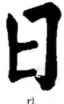

rì

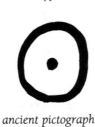

ancient pictograph for rì

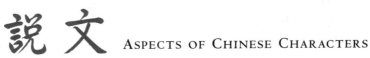 ASPECTS OF CHINESE CHARACTERS

There are several variations of Chinese characters. Perhaps a more accurate way to express this is to say that there are different aspects to Chinese characters. In any given character one or more of these aspects tends to determine its nature. The most common character types belong to one of the categories that follow.

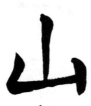 *Pictographs (xiàng xíng)*

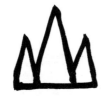

shān

ancient pictograph for shān

These are probably the oldest characters. They are depictions of objects, phenomena, actions, and relationships between things and events. The character for "sun" is a good example of a typical pictograph. The modern character is *rì*. It means "day" but also has other meanings. In its most ancient form it was a simple drawing of the sun, a circle with a dot in its center.

Another example of a typical pictograph is the character that means "mountain," *shān*. It was originally a drawing of three mountain peaks. The later forms of these characters reflect a gradual abstraction that has taken place over time.

Demonstrative characters (zhǐ shì)

Characters of this aspect or class derive their meaning from a particular relationship, generally a spatial one. For instance, the characters *shàng* and *xià* mean "upper" and "lower" respectively. They also have other meanings that evolved from these two fundamental ones. Here, meaning results from the placement of the small strokes. In the character *shàng,* this small stroke is placed above the base of the character, indicating or demonstrating by spatial relationship the sense of "upper." Similarly, with converse significance, the character *xià* has a small stroke below the upper limit of the character, pointing down.

Another example is *rèn,* which also illustrates this way of conveying meaning within the character itself. The character *dāo* means "knife." In the character *rèn,* a dot is placed beside the cutting edge of the knife. Thus, *rèn* means "sharp edge (of a knife)."

shàng

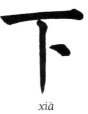

xià

rèn

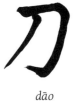

 Ideographs (huì yì)

The difference between pictographs and ideographs is subtle, since both are pictorial representations of objects, phenomena, and their interrelationships. However, ideographs differ from pictographs in that they derive their meaning from the juxtaposition of graphic elements and the images that are thus evoked. The various parts are arranged to evoke the meaning of the ideograph. The character *ān,* described above, is such an ideograph. Another example is the character *míng.* It has many meanings, all of which derive from the juxtaposition of its two radicals. The one on the left is *rì,* sun. The one on the right is *yuè,* moon. The conjunction of the sun and moon elicits the idea of brightness, as both are sources of light. Considering the antiquity of this character, being from an age when there were few if any artificial sources of light, it is clearly a pictorial, albeit abstract, depiction of the idea of "all the light there is." This, indeed, conveys the sense of brightness.

dāo

míng

13

Another example of how this sense is further amplified can be found in one of the many words that is formed with *míng* as an element, "*míng bái*." The character *bái* means "white." Bright and white equate to clear and easy to comprehend. Thus, *míng bái* means "to understand." Another example, embodying what can only be seen as the heroic optimism that has sustained the continuous development of Chinese culture through ten millennia, is the word *míng tiān*. The character *tiān* means "heaven" or "sky." It also means "day," that is, the time during which one sees the sky. Brighter days are certainly what anyone hopes for in the future and "tomorrow" is the meaning of *míng tiān*.

Here then we see several examples of what is meant by the term "ideograph." Ideas depicted by graphic symbols are placed in poignant, abstract relationship so as to evoke meanings that can require many words, even sentences, to completely explain in another language.

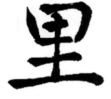

lǐ

A further example of an ideograph that reveals something of how the Chinese language has been formed by the observation of natural phenomena is the character *lǐ*. This character is formed by juxtaposing two other characters. On top is the character *rì*, the sun. Below is the character *tǔ*, the earth. Thus "*lǐ*" is a pictorial representation of the sun moving above the earth. The meaning: the distance that the sun is seen to move across the earth's surface in one hour's time. One *lǐ* is approximately one third of a mile.

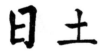

rì   *tǔ*

 Characters whose meanings associate through sound (xíng shēng)

These characters are more complex than the preceding categories. Each single character is comprised of at least two other characters. One represents the sound of the character, another or others signify the meaning. In modern Chinese these account for the vast majority of words. They represent an important step in the development of the language and most resemble the functional characteristics of Western sonographic languages.

WHO CAN RIDE THE DRAGON?

Some scholars propose that Chinese has therefore "outgrown" its ancient tendency to be pictographic and therefore it is erroneous to understand Chinese in terms appropriate to the understanding of pictographs. Regardless of the outcome of this debate, we recognize that the study of the visual roots of the language, as well as all that is implied about the nature and functional habits of those who developed and employed it through the ages, offers us a unique opportunity to gain insight into the Chinese mind. In this context, this category of characters can be understood as the sound-oriented aspect of Chinese.

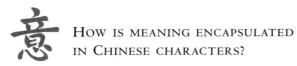 HOW IS MEANING ENCAPSULATED
IN CHINESE CHARACTERS?

This might seem like a strange question. However, it is not so much an inquiry into the philosophy of language as it is a point from which to begin an investigation of the character of the Chinese language and the relationship between the form and content of its words and verbal expressions. If you refer to page 10 and examine the chart comparing the structural organization of Chinese and English, you will see an outline of the formal elements of Chinese. Where Western languages employ a system of sound-encoded, purely abstract forms to convey a particular meaning and encapsulate it in retrievable units, the Chinese have developed an extensive "vocabulary" of representational images which, over millennia, have undergone continual abstraction and simplification. Noticing, like people everywhere, that "a picture is worth a thousand words," the Chinese retained the pictographic nature of their written language and evolved patterns of linguistic operation that included the strong graphic elements essential to a comprehensive understanding of a text.

For our purposes, the important questions are: How does the experience of the Chinese language differ from that of English and other non-Chinese languages? How can someone who knows little if anything about Chinese come to terms with it and learn the knowledge its literature contains? These queries lead to a more general question: How is meaning encapsulated in Chinese characters? This is of particular import when it comes to retrieving meaning from Chinese words and texts, that is, to understanding them. In one sense, Chinese can be understood as a mental or linguistic photography. The characters are visualizations of ideas about things and the ways they act and interact.

These visualizations are made of bits of data (the strokes and radicals) each having discrete meanings or functions. The meanings of the characters are derived from the integration or aggregations of these discrete bits.

One of the first things that we notice when studying Chinese is the fluidity with which one word serves as different parts of speech. The character *shàng* not only means "upper," it also means "go up" or "get on." Thus in Chinese we say *shàng chē* when telling someone to get into a car. To a native English speaker this chameleon nature of Chinese words can be relentlessly disorienting, even distressing, until it becomes familiar. With further study we begin to understand that Chinese is not much concerned with this matter of grammar. The importance of broad, contextual concepts is stressed. This is particularly true in the ancient language, the language of the classical texts of Chinese medicine.

This ancient language was so non-observant of what we know as the basic concepts of modern grammar that it entirely lacked punctuation. In fact, when examining a text written in the ancient language, the first step is to decipher the text's direction of flow. Does it move from left to right, up to down, up to down and left to right across the page, or up to down and right to left across the page? The classical convention was from top to bottom, right to left, thus the "backwards" appearance of Chinese books to non-Chinese. Yet, there are examples of elaborate wordplay—palindromes—in which one text can be read in several directions, each one yielding different, sometimes complementary meanings.

Thus we are well-advised to carefully evaluate any attempt to formulate descriptions of Chinese characters or the language in general, let alone rules about how it functions. In the past, foreign as well as Chinese scholars have exuberantly fallen prey to the temptation to devise eloquent descriptions and patterns to characterize Chinese. The words of Lao Zi from 2500 years ago come to mind: "Beautiful words are not true and truthful words are not beautiful." Chinese is a living, changing language, spoken by over one-quarter of the world's population.

In struggling to develop our own understanding of the language, and particularly how to translate it, we have glimpsed several insights concerning its functional nature. Compared to English, classical or ancient Chinese tends to function more spatially. Where meaning in English unfolds in a linear or temporal mode, Chinese uniquely develops a dimensionality or harmonic of meaning. Again, this is rooted in the pictorial origins of the characters. Though English letters have historical

WHO CAN RIDE THE DRAGON?

roots in Semitic pictographic writing, functionally this aspect of English has completely fallen away. One hundred years ago a theory of the Chinese written character as a medium of poetry was proposed by Ernest Fenellosa and later advanced enthusiastically by the poet Ezra Pound. Recently scholars have tended to repudiate this method of understanding Chinese characters, arguing, for the most part correctly, that modern Chinese people are scarcely aware of the pictorial aspect of their language. Nevertheless, the pictorial roots of the language are still vital and evident in the modern language, to say nothing of a vivid presence in ancient texts. When working to develop an understanding of Chinese medicine, we must particularly consider this characteristic of the Chinese written language.

In this wise, we can trace the roots of comprehensive thinking in Chinese traditional medicine directly back to the natural holism of the Chinese character. We can perceive a Chinese character in much the same way as we perceive a picture or a drawing. It is not a linear, time-bound perception, rather an immediate, dimensional, all-at-once awareness of the thing itself.

A Chinese sentence is composed of a series of such whole images interacting with one another in a multidimensional way to develop clusters of sense and meaning. Thus, much of the classical written language appears as dense, concise expressions that on their surfaces can seem to be trifling aphorisms. But beneath this surface lie variegated regions of meaning and wisdom that require years, indeed decades, of patient study to penetrate and comprehend.

The problem of understanding a single Chinese character can be understood as a microcosm of this same process, although in some cases, a single character can present and represent such an elaborate body of wisdom that the microcosm can take on macrocosmic proportions. The character *dào* 道 is an example of such an intriguingly simple yet ineffable word/concept.

 UNDERSTANDING THE MEANING OF CHARACTERS

How then can we understand the meaning of characters? As with all understanding, familiarity is the fundamental prerequisite. Long before they learn their written language, Chinese children, like children the world over, acquire an understanding of the sounds of words and learn to associate the proper meanings with those sounds. This is accomplished by becoming familiar with the language day by day. When they begin to study the complex and difficult array of written characters, they have a great advantage over anyone who lacks this fundamental familiarity with the words. As they are introduced to new characters, they learn to associate the visual images of the characters with the already familiar sound-meanings they have previously acquired.

Though it is not necessarily true that someone who is familiar with a subject or a character will understand it, familiarity is unequivocally of fundamental importance. Anyone who is unfamiliar with a subject, a word, or a character cannot possibly understand it.

It is important to recognize that a Chinese character conveys its contents within a well-defined visual field. That field consists of several parts or aspects. There is a top, a bottom, a left and right side. The component parts of characters acquire some of their significance from the portion of this visual field they occupy. The process of understanding Chinese characters begins by recognizing their component parts and where they fit in relation to this visual field and in relation to one another.

Character components are subject to morphological changes depending on where they fit in this array of interrelationships. The character for water, *shuǐ*, goes through a distinctive visual alteration when it appears on the left-hand side of compound characters. In such instances it appears as three dots arranged vertically. To signify frozen water, or ice, one of the drops is omitted. Thus some mechanical familiarity is needed to read and understand Chinese characters.

We cannot presume in this book to teach you how to read and understand Chinese. However, by presenting the essential guideposts for reading Chinese we can offer a perspective on the varieties of meaning that Chinese characters may possess. One of the great pitfalls facing

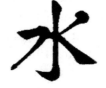

shuǐ

character for water as the left-hand side of a compound character

character for frozen water (ice) as the left-hand side of a compound character

WHO CAN RIDE THE DRAGON?

anyone who translates Chinese, particularly ancient Chinese, into any Western language is that the variable connotations of the characters are too easily rendered as overly simplistic unidimensional ideas. It is as if the original characters enact a field of possible meanings which together portray an overall "meaning" adaptive to any particular context. Yet, when translating this "meaning" into English, much of this multidimensionality can be lost. As we have described, this process of "meaning" begins with the formation of the character from its component parts. It extends through the formation of compound characters and words, and is found in the curious phenomenon of idioms and old sayings.

成 語 IDIOMS AND SAYINGS

Languages and linguistic traditions worldwide possess idiomatic expressions and sayings that convey insights, common knowledge, and collective wisdom distilled from ages of human interaction. Such expressions, often related to myth and folklore, fill the English vernacular. For example, the expression "sour grapes" comes from a fable of Aesop in which the fox, unable to reach the grapes growing overhead, pronounces them sour to assuage his frustration at being unable to taste them. The meaning of the expression, "fool's gold" derives from an effort to describe a natural phenomenon, in this case a mineral that resembles gold in its high degree of reflectivity, yet is far less rare.

In a similar fashion, Chinese speakers rely heavily on pithy expressions from antiquity to communicate their thoughts, impressions, conclusions, and emotions. These sayings are typically concise summations of the essential meaning of ancient stories, in much the same way as we derive the expression "sour grapes." However, there is an intrinsic difference between English and Chinese in how such expressions function within the matrix of their generative language. When approaching Chinese from a Western background and perspective, one of the first and most obvious manifestations of this difference is the frequency with which such expressions appear. This applies to both spoken and written communications.

We offer a simple observation: the Chinese language features a markedly higher degree of dependence on old sayings than does English.

The Language of Chinese Medicine

If we reflect on the reasons for this, we may discover that they illuminate similar trends and tendencies that imbue the constructs and patterns of Chinese medicine.

With this clearly in mind, we note the following:

There is a tendency of the Chinese language, at the level of design and construction of the individual characters, to favor the most concise possible condensation of the sense of a particular object, action, or phenomenon. Albert Einstein said that "everything should be as simple as possible . . . and no simpler." The ancient architects of Chinese may well have had a similar doctrine in mind.

This same tendency is visible even in the more complex strata of the language, and we see it clearly reflected in a reliance upon brief, epigrammatic utterances that contain and convey a wide range of complex emotional and intellectual meanings.

In sum, we might say that Chinese has a predilection for the subtle, the implicit, the unspoken, and the concise. To be sure, it is not a singular predilection, and we can identify an almost opposite one favoring the opulent, the magnificently ornate, and the overwhelmingly grand. These two apparently contrary tendencies do, indeed, exist in China and Chinese both ancient and modern. In fact, a number of such paradoxes present themselves to students of Chinese culture. The cultural landscape is strewn with them. These are the contradictions that merely evoke knowing smiles from those who are questioned.

Beyond knowing smiles, we can also understand several old idiomatic sayings by investigating intrinsic Chinese characteristics such as the love of paradox. This love of paradox is evident in a saying of Mao Ze Dong: "In order to raise fish you must throw a little dung into the water." In authoring countless sayings, Mao was a contemporary exponent of this Chinese tradition of creating epigrammatic expressions to convey a profound intent. Although its contents may have been revolutionary in spirit and intent, the famous *Little Red Book* of quotations from Chairman Mao was traditional in mood, taking its place in a boundless sea of old sayings and quotations from sources famous and infamous throughout history. Here we offer a few examples of such sayings with brief explanations of their origins and meanings.

The expression *"duì niu tán qín"* means literally, "play music to a cow." The story goes like this: One day a young man was playing his *qín*

WHO CAN RIDE THE DRAGON?

(an ancient stringed instrument) in a field. Nearby stood a cow. No matter how beautifully the man played, the cow did not respond. Frustrated that his sole listener found no delight in his music, the young man changed his tune. He played the sound of buzzing flies followed by the sound of a lowing calf. Hearing these sounds, the cow did, indeed, respond, wagging its tail and picking up its ears for further sounds of the calf. It then returned to chewing its cud, indifferent to the musician. Frustrated Chinese school teachers can often be heard repeating this old saying to their inattentive students. "It's like playing music to a cow!"

Another commonly heard expression comes from a story told about the Han Dynasty. A diplomat from the Han court traveled southwest to the ancient kingdom of Yè Láng. There he was received by the local ruler who wanted to know, "Which kingdom is greater, the Han or the Yè Láng?" The diplomat's mettle was tested by this question, since the state of Yè Láng was no larger than a single prefecture of the Han empire. The saying "Yè Láng zì dà" means literally, "Yè Láng has a big impression of itself." It is used to describe people who possess unrealistic images of their own grandeur, comparable to the English saying, "a legend in his own mind."

Still another old saying comes from a fable told in the Western Han Dynasty about a cicada, a praying mantis, a bird, and a young boy. The mantis happened to spy the cicada busily chewing the bark of a tree. He was about to reach out and grab it with his long front legs, but he failed to notice the bird, standing just behind. The bird took advantage of the mantis' preoccupation and was about to nab it with its beak, but it too failed to take note of a young boy hiding behind bushes nearby, the slingshot in his hands aimed right at the bird's head. Táng láng pú chán literally means, "the mantis captures the cicada." This saying is used to describe anyone who fixates only on easily obtained benefits without care or consideration for the dangers or potential loss.

Our final example from among the literally thousands and thousands of such old sayings concerns an old man and a horse that runs away. The old man lived in the north, not far from Mongolia. When the horse disappeared, his neighbors all came round to express their condolences. "We'll see," was all the old man replied. After a few days, the horse came back at the head of a small herd of wild Mongolian ponies. Once again the villagers came round, this time to congratulate the old man on his good fortune. Once again, all the old man would say is, "We'll see." The next day the old man's son went hastily to work breaking-in the new horses, but he carelessly let himself be thrown by a bucking young stallion. The fall broke the young man's leg. When they heard the news, the villagers came round again, offering their expressions of sorrow to the old man for the loss of his son's labor. "We'll see," is all the old man would say. The following day, the imperial army came through town on its way to battle. Every able bodied young man in the village was conscripted and taken away to fight. The villagers returned to congratulate the old man on the great good fortune of having his son left at home, and one more time, all the old man had to say was, "We'll see."

We have heard this story many times. Sometimes it stretches out to episode after episode, the old man's fortunes swaying back and forth from windfall to disaster. The old man, an ardent Daoist, would never reply except with his laconic, "We'll see." The saying *"sài wēng shī mǎ"* literally means "the old man loses his horse." However, it is used to sum the whole flavor of events that taken today as loss result in tomorrow's gain—and vice versa.

This tendency of the Chinese language to condense complex meanings into brief aphorisms appears as a feature of the study and understanding of Chinese medicine. Sayings such as, "*Qì* is the commander of the blood; blood is the mother of *qì*," have been excerpted from ancient sources, in this case the *Yellow Emperor's Canon of Internal Medicine*. These sayings are learned by heart in Chinese medical schools and serve as mnemonic devices for students who must comprehend the abundance of anatomical and physiological data that is thereby implied. Understanding and relating terse expressions to profound, complex, and subtle meanings is thus essential for a student of Chinese medicine. Without such an understanding we would be left with a head full of quaint but virtually meaningless words and phrases. For Chinese students, the task begins with the study of the ancient sources that provide the deeper layers of meaning. But for students of Chinese medicine who have not been raised in the cultural and linguistic environment of China, the work must begin at a different point.

That is, in fact, the point of this entire book; the point at which such work must begin. By investigating the form and function of these old Chinese sayings, readers can understand the material they will encounter as we continue our exploration of the nature and efficacy of Chinese medicine. There is an appropriate old saying often used by those who teach in China. It embodies the hope of teachers that their students might surpass them in understanding and accomplishment: "May the blue of the dye extracted from it be deeper than that of the indigo plant!"

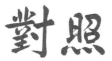 How is Chinese Different from English?

This might seem like a simple question. "Completely!" would be one good answer. It certainly is the most apt answer when a non-native first examines the Chinese language. First impressions, though lasting, can often be misleading. This is not to suggest that Chinese is not completely different from English. It is to suggest, however, that there is something of value to be gained by a more detailed investigation into the several differences that exist between these two languages.

The first of several categories of differences between English and Chinese is origin. First, then, we must ask, what are the origins of the Chinese language? How do they compare to those of English? Next we must pose for ourselves these questions: What are the characteristic ways in which each language develops patterns of thought, logic, and expression? How does the use of Chinese affect and influence the whole experience of those who use it? How does this differ from the ways in which English influences the experience of English speakers?

The several idiosyncrasies of both languages allow us to identify characteristic differences, provide a comprehensive understanding of how Chinese differs from English, and help us compensate for those differences when studying materials and ideas that originate in ancient Chinese. *Vive la difference!* goes the old French saying, and we invoke the wisdom of this advice.

 Origins

Our experience helping Chinese students understand English grammar left a lasting impression, or rather, a lasting series of impressions. Among these, none is clearer than the sudden recognition by Chinese students that, unlike their own language, modern English springs from many different sources. "That explains why the grammar is so complicated," one student remarked after a lengthy discussion of the Greek, Latin, German, French, Spanish, and even Chinese roots of some English words. Looking at this same situation from the opposite viewpoint also offers a useful insight.

The English language is a collection of words and grammar from many linguistic sources. Perhaps this is the reason the study of foreign languages has traditionally played a prominent role in the liberal arts education of Western students. We understand something about our own language by studying foreign languages that share its oldest roots and thus contribute many words, phrases, and grammatical and syntactical patterns. For example, a knowledge of the French influence that followed the Norman conquest in 1066 provides a student of English invaluable information about how English acquired some of its notably French characteristics.

Like England, China has been invaded several times, successfully and unsuccessfully. But a curious result was almost always obtained, at least for roughly the last 2000 years. Those invaders who succeeded in conquering the native Chinese armies quickly adopted Chinese customs, language, and cultural artifacts. Though a statement like this is bound to evoke a lively response from sinologists, we risk and welcome such response to make our point: the Chinese language is derived almost entirely from one source—the Chinese language.

This is not meant to be a mean tautology or worse. One of the characteristic differences between English and Chinese is that where English derives from numerous "parent" languages, Chinese, as it is spoken and used throughout the world today, is almost uniquely derived from its ancient antecedent. Several speculations develop from this fact. Here, however, there is one main area of speculation: How does the uniquely Chinese origin color the nomenclature of Chinese medicine?

In the West we are accustomed to associating Latin words and phrases with medical meanings. Laypeople do not expect to understand the language of medicine as it is used by the specialists with whom they conduct their conventional Western medical affairs. In fact, the entire structure of modern Western education for the past several hundred years has been heavily influenced by Latin. This ancient language is a scientific standard, or perhaps we should say "standard bearer." It does something quite significant to medicine when the doctors who practice it are capable of conversing in an exclusive tongue. By contrast, as we have mentioned above, the language of Chinese medicine is entirely derived from common Chinese words that people have been using for generations. Thus Chinese people have an inherent familiarity with the vocabulary by which they interact with traditional medicine. This is not the case for a non-Chinese individual.

 Patterns of thinking, logic, and expression

One of the most characteristic differences between Chinese and English is the lack of the verb "to be" in common utterances that express what we understand in English to be states of being. "How are you?" "I am fine." Even the contracted "I'm fine" pays full homage to the omnipresent English copula, "to be." The Chinese have a perfectly functional verb "to be." They simply do not use it in the same way, or with the same frequency, as do speakers of English and similar Western languages. This omission of the verb "to be" is representative of a broad tendency in Chinese that might be termed "condensation" or "ephemeralization." Of course to a native user of Chinese, there is no omission. It's just the way that language is. The corresponding view might be expressed by saying how strange it is to Chinese people that English speakers feel the need to state that things are themselves and to express their various states and attributes.

Thus we arrive at an important point. This characteristic way of using the language, this condensation of meanings, reflects a fundamental predilection of the Chinese state of mind. This predilection finds clear expression in an old saying: "One less thing is better than one more thing." Such a remark could be interpreted as the worldview of the shiftless and the idle. No doubt it has been invoked more than once over the centuries to excuse its user from some chore. However, we are not talking about individual people or even populations. We are discussing insights into the collective psyche that have expressed through the span of Chinese history—specifically, those insights gained by careful observation of the language.

Duō yī shì bù rú shǎo yī shì: "One more thing is not as easy as one less thing," is an expression of a deeply rooted Chinese philosophy. It echoes a sentiment that is to be found in the *Dào Dé Jīng*: "To pursue knowledge, gather every day. To pursue the *Dào*, lose every day." We will not be so bold as to identify this tendency any further.

The paradigm of this sort of cultivation of the intellectual as well as the spiritual self can be found in the Confucian classic, *Dà Xué* (*The Great Learning*). In this work, a long recipe for self-cultivation expands to include the provision of both an orderly household and a well-governed state:

> *[Self-cultivation] . . . is rooted in sorting things into organic categories. When things had been classified in organic categories, knowledge moved toward fulfillment; given the extreme knowable points, the inarticulate thoughts were defined with precision [the sun's lance coming to rest on the precise spot verbally]. Having attained this precise verbal definition [lit: this sincerity], they then stabilized their hearts; they disciplined themselves; having attained self-discipline, they set their own houses in order; having order in their own homes, they brought good government to their own states; and when their states were well governed, the empire was brought into equilibrium.*

The text goes on to identify "self-discipline" as the root. For our present purpose, however, we focus on the phrase, "the inarticulate thoughts were defined with precision" because it is this phrase that we have referred to as a paradigm for a broader tendency of the Chinese language, the Chinese cultural state of mind.

The ancient Chinese language is an extraordinarily dense woven tapestry of words and ideas. It is as if the enormous mass of century upon century of literary endeavor functioned like the mass of a star, compressing the component elements ever more tightly together to change, compress, and condense their essential nature. The resulting core glows brightly with enormous energy: there are voluminous packets of information that thus distilled and refined are capable of transmitting their fascinating, curious, and often esoteric contents far into the unknown space of the future. Here today, we have received a large transmission from this steadily accumulating cultural object that we identify as Chinese traditional medicine. By examining and understanding its materials, we can illuminate whole vistas of knowledge and wisdom that lie within the territory bounded by these words.

Another fascinating pattern of the Chinese language is to be found in the syntax for asking questions. Questions reflect the way we gather information about the world. For instance, the typical questions we pose

WHO CAN RIDE THE DRAGON?

in English to "find out all about" some thing or matter are "Who?" "What?" "Where?" "When?" and "Why?" This fairly casual observation actually imparts some information about the mental predilections of those who proceed to gather information with these questions.

The Chinese have a characteristic way of asking a question. It is to make a statement and then pose its negative as an alternative. For example, "How are you doing?" translates into Chinese as, "*Ní hǎo bù hǎo.*" Literally these words mean, "You good not good?" Similarly, a common way of asking someone whether they would like to go somewhere is, "*Zóu bù zóu?*" or, in literal translation, "Go not go?"

This "positive-negative" question formation is both prevalent in and characteristic of the way Chinese people use their language. It is far more prevalent among Chinese than the typical American uses of the same sentence structure. "You going or not?" is the type of sentence you might use to lend force or stress to the issue. But in Chinese, this is just as common, perhaps the most common, way to formulate questions. It reflects a set of fundamental intellectual or cultural considerations. These can be summed under the heading of primitive dialectics, the type that gave rise to yīn-yáng theory.

The traditional Chinese view sees the world as the result of the interplay of fundamental forces, powers, or energies. It is reflected in the way Chinese ask questions, and in the way they tend to understand the answers to those questions. We have often received, with a sort of curious bemusement, answers from various teachers as to the difference between related concepts. "What is the difference between the blood and the *qì*?" asks the ingenuous student. "Blood is blood; *qì* is *qì*," comes the response. We sense at such times that the meaning is deeper than the surface appearance. In truth it is. It is the light that shines from the fire of the philosophical and spiritual wisdom compressed into the ideas of *qì* and blood through Chinese history.

We want a feeling for the language sensitized by identifying characteristic patterns that can serve as touchstones. Lacking this "feeling" severely limits our ability to take hold of the meaning of words. Rooted in the concrete, graphic nature of Chinese words, there is an intuitive, immediate sense or understanding that must be evoked to appreciate the overall communications of the Chinese written word—or speech for that matter. This immediacy of the language is not altogether different from similar phenomena in other tongues. Again, the point is to identify how such phenomena occur in the hands and on the tongues of Chinese writers, thinkers, teachers, and doctors.

One of the curious features that seems to accompany notions of textual literary interpretation in the Chinese tradition is that the intellect as well as the emotional content of the readers' or interpreters' mind must, as a matter of implicit importance, be a dynamic part of the development of the "meaning" of the text investigated. This is almost a paraphrase of a principle that arose in Western science with the ascendancy of quantum mechanics, to wit: the act of observation impinges upon, in fact profoundly alters, the object or phenomenon that is being observed. It is as if the Chinese have known this through the course of their 5000-year history of writing and reading, collecting and passing on all their great works of the literary and scientific arts. Naturally, the meaning of these words will change as they find their ways into various minds in various times and places. Thus we see conventions of linguistic use, patterns of how the language operates, accruing still another important role in the overall process of transmission of information from century to century and millennium to millennium.

This concerns what we might refer to as "mnemonic devices." Imagine, for instance, that you are a librarian who must deal with 5000 years worth of entries in your catalog. You, as well as your ancestors, absolutely must have a shorthand for dealing with the masses of data that accumulate over such a span. The essence of such shorthand devices are to be found in the classical literature itself.

One typical pattern is that of the "three-word canon." There is a work like this in nearly every field of endeavor, especially those that possess ancient roots. In short, a *sān zì jīng* is a collection of lines, easily committed to memory, that contain a wide variety of rhyme, rhythm, and other mnemonic devices to help students and other users learn and remember for future use. This approach to communicating information is nothing new in China. The sing-song repetition of lessons in Chinese schools at virtually every grade from elementary school to college is in no way an invention of the Communist regime. It reflects something old and basic about how Chinese learn to obtain information. It is, as we note, rooted in the language patterns themselves and reflected in many ways in a course of traditional subjects.

WHO CAN RIDE THE DRAGON?

Why? One answer can be found in the traditional concept of *gōng fū*. What is *gōng fū*? It is the skill that develops, in time, through strenuous labor. This implies rigorous repetition of drills, both verbal and physical. In Chinese traditional subjects, in the Chinese way of looking at skill to evaluate it, no *gōng fū* means no skill. If you have not invested taxing hours of labor in study and practice, you cannot expect to achieve anything at all. This goes far beyond a basic concept like "work hard and you will be rewarded." It verges on the mysterious in terms of traditional subjects like *qì gōng, tài jí quán,* and other arts that train the breath and develop *gōng fū* concerning the body's most fundamental energies.

Gōng fū is reflected in the very nature of the language itself, in how it is used, and in the patterns that become recognizable as familiarity with Chinese words and their curious contents develops. When a person of learning writes with the brush, his or her entire life, their whole collection of skill and understanding, is reflected in a single stroke, in the appearance of single dot. The Chinese language encourages us to look for and find meaning everywhere, in every breath, every utterance, every mark left by those who took the time to speak, write, or otherwise record their thoughts.

Those that have survived the test of time proceed into the future, the sum total of the considered experience of a people. By coming to terms with some basic ways in which this continuous progression of language and literary tradition moves, we aim to provide readers with greater access to the contents, the meanings of the words, the texts, and the ideas that give them vitality.

風格 *Idiosyncrasies*

An idiosyncrasy is a peculiar habit or mannerism. Here we use it to refer to a habit and mannerism of language that does not seem to fit the other categories of our discussion. There are, indeed, such mannerisms of language and, in comparing those of English with those of Chinese, it is possible to further understand the way meaning is transmitted in both languages. Importantly, this process of comparison can also help us take meanings from one (Chinese) and bring them into the other (English), alive and in working order.

Earlier, we mentioned the tendency of the Chinese language to favor brevity in verbal expressions. As we have pointed out, one of the idiosyncratic features that reflects this tendency is the fluid, at times nearly amorphous nature of what we know in English as "parts of speech." A typical Chinese word frequently functions as noun, verb, and modifier during the course of everyday use. To non-native learners of the language, this chameleon-like quality can be particularly troublesome, for Chinese words do not undergo any change in form or sound relative to their variable use in different contexts.

This leads to another characteristic of the Chinese language which could be termed contextual dependency. What a Chinese word means, at any point, depends heavily on context. This is true grammatically, in determining a word's role in a sentence as a particular part of speech, but it is no less true in terms of compositional style. This requires that students of the Chinese language, and of those subjects that are primarily transmitted by language, possess an enormous familiarity with the possible contexts.

In essence, that is why we wrote this book, to introduce how the Chinese language and traditional subjects go about cultivating and transmitting meaning and knowledge. Just as over one thousand years ago Sun Si Miao emphasized that a well-trained doctor must possess a familiarity with many subjects and schools of thought, Western students of Chinese medicine are no less subject to the same requirements, regardless of what local governing agencies may establish as the legal guidelines for licensure. Indeed, they face the even more onerous task of first recognizing that such requirements exist. Once we accept this fact, we can begin to explore ways to gain access to these vast fields and to begin the lifelong process of finding meaning and cultivating understanding and wisdom.

Chinese scholars from antiquity to the present have understood this as a context-dependent activity; it can only be accomplished by an individual within the limits of his or her own understanding of the ideas and precepts. What are these ideas? We have tried to distill an irreducible minimum, as listed in the Table of Contents. To appreciate the importance of this sensitivity to context, we need to grasp that it is hard-wired into the language itself.

By growing up speaking, reading, and writing Chinese, an individual naturally develops a sense of how meanings are constellated, how shorthand references to huge bodies of thought are accomplished with a single word, and, of vital importance, how to go about navigating by such lights. It is important to recognize such habits in trying to approximate a native understanding.

For the Chinese, the mood of a sentence, established through the use of particular words, is more important than what is known in English as "tense" or the time factor. Just as they undergo no change in form or sound to express their function as different parts of speech, Chinese words, particularly verbs, do not undergo any morphological change to denote different tenses. For example, the word *liǎo* conveys a sense of something that is already completed. The word *zhe* conveys the mood of actions that continue or are progressive. To be sure, the Chinese talk about the past, present, and future, but references to these distinctions are not accomplished in the same fashion as they are in English. We might conclude that Chinese people have a different sense of themselves in time than do users of English.

Yet such idiosyncratic differences are merely reflections of a basic divergence that does indeed exist between Chinese and English. The best way to illustrate this is to present several examples of problems facing those who translate ancient Chinese concepts into modern English.

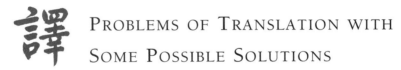

PROBLEMS OF TRANSLATION WITH SOME POSSIBLE SOLUTIONS

It is the aim of this book to help readers develop an understanding of Chinese medicine as well as a methodology for comprehending it in its cultural context. In Chapter 7, you will find a list of one hundred or more words and terms that form the essential nomenclature of the subject. For now, we hope that by providing extended explorations of the following three basic concepts—*shū xué*, *qì*, and *yīn-yáng*— we can suggest ways you can study and understand the material more fully.

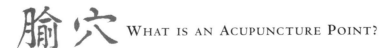

WHAT IS AN ACUPUNCTURE POINT?

In Chinese medical nomenclature, there is some confusion as to the names of acupuncture points. This applies to the general term for acupuncture point as well as to the names of specific points. This reflects the general, inherent ambivalence of the terminology of Chinese medicine.

In fact, no one really knows what an acupuncture point is. This is not to say that there is not a body of information concerning acupuncture points, their nature, structure, function, interrelationships, and interactions. Indeed there is an abundance of such accumulated knowledge and experience from thousands of years of using acupoints to treat illness. Nevertheless, the most reliable authorities in Chinese medicine seem to agree that there is something mysterious about acupuncture points. Indeed, much of Chinese medicine is rooted in concepts and methods of thought that are shadowy, elusive, and difficult to discuss. This does not forbid discussion, but informs us when we enter into one.

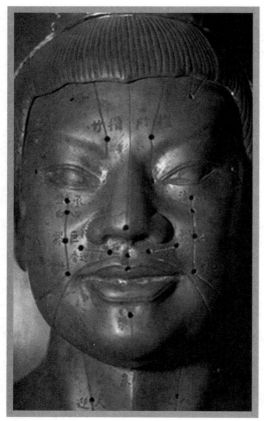

Acupuncture points on the famous bronze model from the Song Dynasty

An acupuncture point is a component of a system. Acupuncture points possess a reflexive characteristic in relation to this system. They seem to be, and to function as, micro-mirrors of the body. In Chinese medicine, the body is considered to be a microcosm of the entire universe. Thus acupuncture points have a peculiarly complex nature.

What do they reflect? In essence, they reflect information, energy, states of being, conditions of existence of the body and the mind, of the being as a whole, and its component parts. The system that comprises the acupuncture points is likewise a reflexive system of information generation and conveyance. In traditional Chinese medicine this system is known as *jīng luò*. It is usually translated into English as either "meridians" or "channels and network vessels."

WHO CAN RIDE THE DRAGON?

The Chinese character *jīng* has many meanings: to manage or deal in; constant, regular; canon (as in the sense of a classic work in a literary tradition); to pass through; as a result of. It is also part of a considerable number of words that have an even wider variety of meanings. With relation to the system of which the acupuncture points are components, we can probably best understand the meaning of *jīng* as "to pass through" or "thoroughfare."

jīng

The word *luò* is somewhat simpler. It means anything resembling a net; to tie or to wind. It signifies the action and result of weaving together as a net or mesh. Thus the system of acupuncture points can be visualized as a matrix that passes through the body, connecting all of its parts and serving as an energy/communications grid that generates, propagates, stores, and releases information and force related to the body and its various components. It is a comprehensive system, a descriptor of the whole body. Every place in the body is permeated by and connected with every other place in the body by means of the *jīng luò* system. In short, it is the fundamental infrastructure of Chinese anatomy and physiology. Importantly, this system also serves to connect the body to the environment, providing access between the body—both in terms of various body surfaces as well as the internal organs—and environmental influences, energies, and information.

luò

The Chinese word-concept that we translate into English as "acupuncture point" is composed of elements conveying the sense of "body transport (or communications) hole." It is written *shū xué*. The first character, *shū*, is composed of several elements. The left-hand side is the radical that means "flesh," 月 *rù*. It appears in numerous words related to the body, body parts, and organs. The right-hand side is the character *shū* 俞, which in turn is made up of four radicals. The top-most is the radical for person, *rén* 人. Beneath this radical is the radical *yī* 一, which means "one." Beneath this there are two additional radicals. On the left is, again, the flesh radical, 月 *rù*. On the right is the radical *dāo* 刂, which means knife.

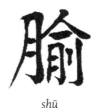

shū

The Language of Chinese Medicine

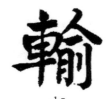

shū

This character is closely related in form and meaning to another that is frequently used to describe acupuncture points and which, in ancient times, was frequently interchanged with *shū* in written texts. Though pronounced the same, the difference between the two is that the left-hand side of *shū* is the radical that means vehicle or transportation. Thus the sense of transportation is involved in the overall meaning of the word.

By a linguistic process of borrowing or sharing meaning between two otherwise unrelated words, this sense of transportation is also included in the character *shū*. The character *shū* is usually used to refer to a special group of points located on the back that are particularly involved in the movement of the *qì* of the various internal organs. The general meanings of these two characters have grown closely together over the centuries of development of Chinese medicine.

xué

The second character in the word *shū xué* is *xué*. The top part, as mentioned above, represents a roof or covering and is frequently seen in characters related to dwelling places. The bottom part signifies dividing; it also means the numeral eight. The literal interpretation of this character could be "a dwelling place that results from dividing (or opening up)." It is commonly translated into English as "cave, hole, or crevice." In informal usage and spoken (rather than written) language, acupuncture points are often referred to as *xué wèi*. The second character, *wèi*, means simply "place" or "location."

Functionally, acupuncture points seem to have two most basic actions: they open and they close. The names of many points include words that mean gate, pass, or door. In opening, they release information and energy. In closing, they store it. In that sense, they can be understood to function like a capacitor in an electric circuit. In therapeutic use, we might liken them to a transducer. They are places where the mechanical energy of the needle is transformed into energy and information that the body can understand and use to balance itself. Such

WHO CAN RIDE THE DRAGON?

comparisons are of limited value, as capacitors and transducers are precisely rated devices where acupuncture points seem to be more or less randomized in terms of their various capacities. This randomization occurs between individuals, that is, the same point on different individuals cannot be expected to possess the same capacity for information or energy storage or conveyance. It also occurs in the same individual with changes in time, location, environmental conditions and influences, and internal body states.

The acupuncture points are dynamic elements; they are always changing. To understand them more fully, one must investigate their individual locations, functions, and applications in the treatment of diseases and conditions of the body/mind. In clinical use, they represent the thoroughfares through which the doctor can influence the patient's condition. In simple terms, the doctor is restoring the balance of fundamental processes within the patient, based on the Chinese traditional medical theories which are discussed elsewhere in detail.

Bearing in mind the above description, that the points themselves possess the potential of opening and closing like gates, we can get a basic idea of how the doctor proceeds. Guided by theory, the doctor first assesses the patient's condition, comprehending the state of the body and its various parts. These theories provide the skilled and knowledgeable doctor with a basis for anticipating and determining the condition of the individual acupoints, which might be closed, requiring opening or vice versa. This can also be thought of as "draining" or "supplementation." This is an oversimplification, but the principle inheres in what the doctor is doing.

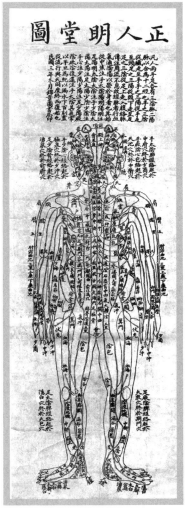

A 1914 chart
showing an anterior view
of the circulation of qì through the
channels and network vessels

35

The Language of Chinese Medicine

A doctor observing a certain pattern of conditions in a patient need not look everywhere in the body for acupoints to treat. The doctor is guided by theory to specific points. Then, by applying further theories and techniques, he or she assesses the accuracy of this initial judgment and locates the right points to treat at that specific time. Essentially, we find these points in various states of opening, closing, failing to open, failing to close. That portion of the system of channels and network vessels, represented and interrelated to the various points, is correspondingly replete or vacuous. Replete or vacuous of what? The answer can be simply stated, but it is difficult to grasp the deeper meaning.

The channels contain and convey *qì* and blood (*xuè*). These words require thorough investigation before they can be fully understood. Then, again in simple terms, the physician performs various needle manipulations designed to open points that are pathologically closed and vice versa. One can visualize the acupuncture points as diaphragms (for example, the diaphragm in a camera lens) that regulate the amount of energy/information moving along these pathways at particular locations throughout the body.

The theory of the channels and network vessels provides a comprehensive map of the body, marked in hundreds of places with acupoints that have specific functions in relation to the organs, bodily structures, and other points of the body. Thousands of years of clinical experience with these theories has led to the development of an enormous body of data regarding the effects and effectiveness of each of these points for treating patterns of disease and overall conditions of the body/mind. This system is complete in that it correlates the entire body and a comprehensive range of conditions. Yet the essential structure of Chinese medical theory also includes the practitioner's understanding and intuition. It is therefore an open system inviting continual development and refinement.

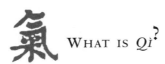 WHAT IS *Qì*?

The apparently simple question, "What is *qì*?" is perhaps the best example of the subtle yet complex difficulties faced when trying to understand and translate basic Chinese medical terms into English. It also clearly illustrates one of the central reasons for this book, namely that without grasping something of the nature of the cultural background of Chinese medicine, we can neither understand nor apply its theories and methods.

The word *qì* is a common component of many words in Chinese. Of course, most of these words have nothing to do with Chinese medicine. *Qì* is also a basic concept in many different disciplines of traditional Chinese culture such as martial arts, *qì gōng,* calligraphy, and painting. In fact, *qì* is one of the most basic concepts in all of Chinese culture. Anywhere you look in Chinese culture, you are likely to encounter the word *qì.* Its meanings may differ; its implications in arts and sciences may be widely variable; yet its presence is constant.

In Chinese folklore, *qì* occurs in the very earliest stories of the creation of the world. (See Chapter 2 for further discussion of this topic.) In fact, to the traditional Chinese mind, everything that exists is *qì* in some form or another. Yet, most would agree that *qì* has no specifically material nature. What is this mysterious substance that is not substance and that functions within and without every phenomena, known and yet to be known, in the universe?

In our search for an answer, a good starting point is an examination of the character itself. This character was originally ≋, a pictograph representing the vapor that rises to form a cloud. In a work called *Bǔ Cí Qiú Yì,* the scholar Yu Shen Wu wrote that this character was easy to confuse with the character for the number three, *sān,* written 三. Thus, as early as the Zhou Dynasty, the character *qì* commenced a long, slow transformation as seen in the illustrations at right.

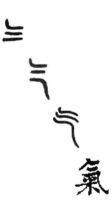

transformations of the character "qì"

The process we have mentioned of borrowing or sharing between unrelated words is involved in the development of the meaning of *qì.* From earliest times, *qì* was associated with the idea of *yún qì* or "cloud *qì,*" that is, the steam that rises from the earth to form the clouds. Another character with which *qì* was associated is *xì.* This character means to give or take, especially to give or take food, to nourish. There are examples in ancient texts of the character *qì* being used in place of *xì* to convey this idea of nourishment. Thus the concept of supporting life came to be associated with the character *qì*.

Another important association with the character *qì* is the concept of *yuán qì* or "original *qì*." In Chinese medicine, this term has a specific meaning which is described in detail in the last chapter. In Chinese culture generally, the *yuán qì* refers to the state of the cosmos before the universe or any matter, energy, space, or time were created. *Yuán qì* is described as being not clear, like a heavy fog. It was conceived of as incomprehensibly dense, so small it could not be seen. Yet it contained the whole of creation that was to come. Eventually, this singularity separated into two aspects. The heavy aspect settled downward, becoming the earth; while the lighter part rose to become the heavens. This is the original separation of yīn and yáng.

With this separation came the existence of *yáng qì*, the pure, light aspect of *yuán qì* that rose to form the heavens. *Yīn qì*, which was the heavy, substantial aspect that settled to become the earth, also appeared. In essence, this is the description of the birth of yīn and yáng. Thus *qì* came to be understood as the most basic element of all things in existence.

The basic nature of *qì* is therefore the manifestation of transformation such as the one that yields steam from water. *Qì* is considered to have two essential characteristics, *yīn qì* and *yáng qì*. These two further subdivide according to the principles of yīn and yáng. *Qì* is not so much a substance as it is the transformative manifestations of processes in nature. Yet it is clear in its derivation that the concept of *qì* includes a substantial aspect, although this substantive nature is ephemeral, indeed, being likened to the vapor that forms the clouds.

One important thing to recognize about the word *qì* is that to the Chinese, *qì* is a vital component of everything. In fact, it is not an overstatement to say that, from the traditional Chinese viewpoint, everything that is sensed or experienced is a manifestation, a form of *qì*. Certainly, this order of importance pertains to the Chinese medical concept of *qì*. A doctor of Chinese medicine is first and last concerned with the patient's *qì*. Does it move naturally, properly? Are the yīn and yáng aspects properly balanced? In other words, is the patient in good health? For health is conceived of as nothing, if it is not the balance of yīn and yáng as manifest by the free-flowing, harmonious circulation of *qì* throughout the patient's body/mind and life.

WHO CAN RIDE THE DRAGON?

Of course, there is much, much more that has been and could be said about *qì*. In the last chapter of this book, the various aspects of *qì* within the body are discussed from the point of view of their meaning in Chinese medicine.

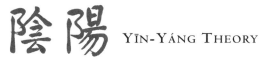 YĪN-YÁNG THEORY

Yīn-yáng theory is one of the oldest doctrines in Chinese culture and one of the most typically Chinese. Its origins are obscured by their antiquity. The words *yīn* and *yáng* were originally pictographic representations of the shady and sunny sides, respectively, of a mountain or hill. They came to represent two primordial forces that were the fundamental constituents of the universe and everything in it. As such, they formed the basic element of an indigenous Chinese naturalistic philosophy that predated the philosophy known as Daoism and which served as the essential seed of Daoist as well as other typically Chinese concepts.

Yīn and yáng were well-developed concepts in the oldest known Chinese text, the *Yì Jīng (I Ching)*. Their most simple and immediate representation is in the diagram known as *tài jí tú*. Successive generations of Chinese thinkers have elaborated a comprehensive description of the cosmos and of human affairs based upon these two concepts. Yet, while amassing a copious literature on the subject, scholars and writers have tended to avoid hard and fast definitions of yīn and yáng. What confronts us in these ancient (as well as contemporary) works are expressions of mystery, wonder, and at times a religious reverence for these two principles. Nonetheless, to grasp the theoretical structure of Chinese medicine, we must grapple with their meanings, for the entire treasurehouse of Chinese medicine is constructed on the foundation of yīn-yáng theory.

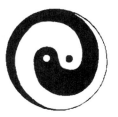

tài jí tú

If we pose the question, "What is *qì*?" Some will answer that it is the result of the interplay between yīn and yáng. Yīn and yáng mix together and *qì* issues forth. Perhaps it is better to say that when yīn and yáng were separated from the singularity at the beginning of existence, the resulting potential gave rise to *qì*. If we next pose the question, "What is the overall purpose of a doctor of Chinese medicine?" many will respond that it is to balance yīn and yáng. A physician must restore this balance when it has been disturbed and must guide patients towards a way of life that maintains this balance.

The concept of mystery lies at the heart of yīn-yáng theory. The mystery of yīn and yáng could be called the heart that beats in the breast of Chinese medicine's body. The Daoist classic, *Dào Dé Jīng*, states, in terms that reflect the mystical mathematics of ancient China:

dào shēng yī	*Dao gives birth to one;*
yī shēng èr	*one gives birth to two;*
èr shēng sān	*two gives birth to three;*
sān shēng wàn wù	*three gives birth to the ten thousand things [everything]*

Yīn and yáng are frequently described as opposites or complementary opposites. In terms of Western thought, however, the notion of opposing forces is a powerful one, echoing in religious, moral, and ethical concepts of right and wrong, good and evil. We therefore must tread lightly when making comparisons between these Western paradigms and the doctrine of yīn and yáng. Although it is true that yīn and yáng are conceived of as being in opposition, this describes just one aspect of their complex pattern of interrelationship. They nourish and foster the growth of one another; they restrain each other; they support one another; they penetrate each other; they always and only co-exist. To simply state that they are opposing forces of nature neglects the importance of their other manifold interactions.

When questioning teachers about the subject, students often experience frustration with the answers. As they study longer and deeper, students develop a growing sense that the more they know about yīn and yáng, the less they can say. There is, perhaps, endless information that could be presented about yīn and yáng. But in the end we will simply recall the words of Lǎo Zǐ:

Dào kě dào fēi cháng dào	*The Dao that can be described as Dao is not the eternal Dao*

The name we can know is not its eternal name. Those who wish to delve deeper into the mysteries of yīn and yáng will find the way difficult but the journey rewarding.

CHAPTER TWO

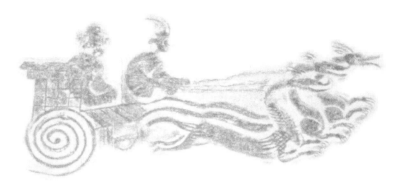

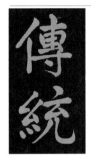

Folk Beliefs, Myths, and Customs

We are the children of the Dragon.

—Old Chinese saying

In the beginning was the word.

—*The Book of Genesis*

WHAT DO WE REALLY KNOW about ancient people and their traditional beliefs and practices? All that can be known is contained in stories, both written and oral, that have survived, providing us glimpses and impressions. Written records are somewhat more accessible than folklore, and we discuss various aspects of the literary tradition in the transmission of ancient knowledge in Chapter Four.

In exploring beliefs, myths, and customs, what we seek are clues as to how the Chinese people have answered the most basic questions of life. Who are we? Where do we come from? What are we doing here? Where are we headed? Such questions and their answers form the basis of every peoples' folklore.

One of the problems encountered in studying this material is in misidentifying ideas because we assume that they are equivalent to ideas in our own cultural context. We think, for example, that the Chinese concept of *qì* must refer to something basic and universal. Propelled by this assumption we stride forth to discover equivalent or analogous concepts in our own heritage. The problem is that we find them, whether or not they exist.

This might seem a peculiar assertion. Yet, in fact, something like this has occurred with *qì*. Many have undertaken to render the word, and various texts describe it, its cultivation, and its role in Chinese medicine and martial arts, as similar or analogous to ideas drawn from the Western frame of reference.

Our approach is diametrically opposed. We begin with the assumption that *qì*, like many other basic ideas and concepts in Chinese medicine, is unique and unparalleled among Western ideas. This is not to say that these ideas are unknowable to Westerners. In fact, they are no less knowable to people in the West than to people in China—even Chinese students must study diligently to understand *qì*. Nevertheless, Chinese students do not face the considerable pitfall of identifying *qì* with words that have little or nothing to do with its traditional nature and function.

Hence we have adopted this posture in order to avoid such a pitfall. We do so not simply because we wish to celebrate Chinese medicine and culture, but also because it succeeds. It succeeds by identifying differences and providing access to new intellectual territory. For those who might have already obtained access to the great treasurehouse of Chinese medicine, we hope to provide further illumination.

There are numerous similarities among the various traditional arts and disciplines of ancient China. We could describe these similarities in various ways, but have chosen to adopt an "organic" method, sorting these similarities into categories that represent the core of the ingredients common to most Chinese cultural manifestations. These are the shared ideas of which culture in China seems to be an expression.

This set of common elements, taken as a whole, is the "root" or living essence of culture in China. To a great extent this root is synonymous with the concept of *qì*. The material in the following sections represents its branches. By examining the branches and tracing the flow of *qì* as it interconnects, we can gain awareness of the root. This awareness is indispensable to understanding the basis of Chinese medicine, for, as Confucius wrote in *The Great Learning*, "If the root be in confusion, nothing will be well-governed."

上古　THE ANCIENT MAGIC WORLD

Long before the conventions of recording history existed, long before any practical technology for recording thoughts or words came into being, in the distant mists of prehistory, Chinese cultural images were already well formed. We once met an archaeologist studying pre-Shang (pre-1600 B.C.E.) bones with hieroglyphic inscriptions. "I like this ancient stuff," he explained over a beer on the balcony of Chengdu's now-defunct but once-famous Reggae Bar, "because I don't have to mess with language. There are no words ... just objects and pictures."

What these pictures convey is an image of a primitive, primordial, and powerful world. It was a world in which spirits and demons freely interacted with human beings, a world where there was no distinct barrier between humankind and nature. Ancient Chinese people conceived of themselves as minions of the natural world in which they lived. They were buffeted by myriad natural and supernatural forces locked in endless and cyclical struggle. Some were far more potent than man, some were within human control, some were misleadingly calm and quiet, then suddenly overpowering and deadly.

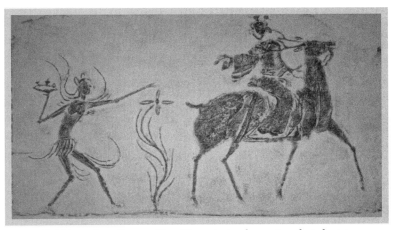

Rubbing taken from a Han Dynasty tomb carving that depicts
a wū (shaman) preparing an herbal medication
for a prince (the soul) to assist his journey

In this ancient past, a group of people, both men and women, were believed to possess special powers enabling them to intervene between

wū

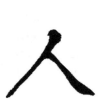

rén

gōng

*early pictograph
of male wū (xí)*

*early pictograph
for wū*

humans, spirits, gods, and demons. The Chinese called such people *wū*. This word can be translated by several English words, each of which captures some but not all the meaning implicit in the Chinese word. As is frequently the case, it takes several sentences to convey the meaning of a single character. They could be called "magicians," "sorcerers," "witches," "warlocks," "necromancers," or other similar names.

An investigation into the character *wū* reveals something of the nature and function of those who bore the name. It consists of the character *gōng*, which means "work," plus the character *rén*, repeated on each side of *gōng*. There were two characters, the one above used to indicate a female *wū*, and another used to denote a male *wū*. The character for a male *wū* included *jiàn*, the character that means "to see." In both characters the upper horizontal stroke, as in many characters, can be understood to mean that which is above, that is, the sky, or heaven. The lower horizontal stroke can be seen as that which is below, the earth. The "sum" of the character can thus be expressed as "two people working to connect heaven and earth." According to China's oldest dictionary, the *Shuō Wén Jiě Zì*, the character evolved from a depiction of an ancient long-sleeved dance, which symbolized the dance rituals performed by these ancient healers when they "worked."

The realm of humanity lies between heaven and earth, and the *wū* could communicate with unseen spirits in the heavens, on earth, or in people's bodies. They interpreted their movements and changes. Thus, as civilization developed, the *wū* became extraordinarily influential. Institutions of power evolved, and kings and emperors were reluctant to act without the advice of their magicians and spiritual guides. They asked about war-making and military strategy. They sought guidance for developing civilization. They followed their advice on issues large and small, down to what clothes to wear on a particular day or whether or not it was wise to go out at all.

Who Can Ride the Dragon?

Clearly, these ancient necromancers played several roles in the lives of the ancient Chinese. They were oracles, sages, and judges, as well as healers. They were the holders of wisdom, those whose power transcended the mundane. People entrusted their health, their fate, their very lives to them. In short, they were China's original doctors at a time when the technology of Chinese medicine was in its infancy. The *wū* were perceived to possess the power to mitigate the influences that resulted in disease as well as other forms of suffering, and were thus also called *wū yī*, the word *yī* meaning "medicine" or "doctor."

The *wū* depended on the power implicit in objects, words, and humans; they depended on the forces of nature to heal. They chanted, danced, and pleaded with evil spirits to leave a diseased patient alone; they scared away the devils that brought disease by uttering potent secret words. They were conduits for influences beyond the understanding or control of man, standing between the people and natural and supernatural forces, which were hardly differentiated in prehistoric times.

These ancient doctors drew upon the implicit power of words to perform their magic medicine. Word magic was an important part of the repertoire of these earliest doctors in China. Traditions of word magic are in no way unique to China, yet in China traditions of word magic are particularly powerful. This stems from the nature of the language itself, the role that words play and the way they are used to capture and crystallize information. Knowledge is power, after all. Through the ages, literacy, the ability to manipulate language to one's own purposes, has been extremely important in Chinese culture, a fact still reflected in Chinese peoples' admiration of poets and scholars.

The roots of Chinese medicine grow in a soil that is dense and darkly matted with primitive traditions, superstitious understandings, and misunderstandings of the natural world and man's role within it. Yet, over the centuries, these primitive fears and confusions were refined and molded into clear and extraordinarily clever perceptions of the forces at work in the three realms of heaven, earth, and humankind. What emerged as a primary aim of medical practitioners was the establishment of harmony between these three realms.

Chinese medicine remains intimately linked to its most ancient roots. Its theories embrace primitive understandings and harness their considerable potentials. They form a pragmatic, highly effective body of knowledge, congealed over the course of centuries, that utilizes techniques for tending to the health of human beings. Literally and figuratively, it arose from ancient mists described by the Chinese as *qì,* and from its source in Chinese mythologies of the world's creation.

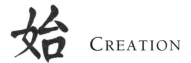

CREATION

Just as a child yearns to know, "Where did I come from?" so do cultures around the world. Each has a traditional explanation, and stories of creation are found in every culture. As these traditions grow and gather momentum, they fortify their hegemony by establishing a pedigree, a chain of ancestors. Among religious traditions this pedigree invariably serves as a link to the immortal, the eternal, the heavenly. Thus, believers are provided an explanation that answers the questions "Where?" "When?" and "Why?" by relation to a unique, original creation.

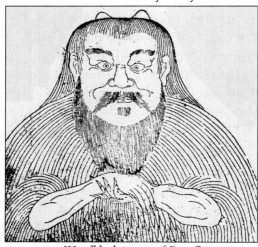

Woodblock image of Pán Gŭ by San Ts'ai T'u Hui (1628-1644), courtesy of Harvard-Yenching Library, Harvard University

The Chinese possess many such myths and tales. Probably the most common and the most Chinese of these tales is the story of Pán Gŭ. We retell it here as it has been handed down since ancient times.

Before the beginning, everything was packed inside a giant egg. The entire cosmos, all matter, energies, spaces, time, numbers— all was stuffed inside this egg. It was packed so tightly that everything was inseparable. It would not have been possible to differentiate any one thing from any other.

The name given to the substance that filled this egg is *yuán qì.* This word has several renderings in English reflecting its several meanings in Chinese language and medicine. Its root meaning, however, is "original *qì.*"

Also inside the egg was the giant, Pán Gŭ. Being in a state before anything existed, when there was nothing except the egg and Pán Gŭ, the giant become bored, impatient, frustrated. He cracked the egg. First an arm appeared, then a leg, then another arm and another leg, and the baby giant Pán Gǔ was born, founding a lineage destined to become nothing less than the people who tell his story.

As he stood among the shards of the cracked egg and the escaping *yuán qì*, something new began to happen. The original *qì* began to separate. Its lighter element rose and formed Heaven. Its heavy and dense aspects sank and formed Earth, and Pán Gǔ stood astride Heaven and Earth. Where he walked, valleys were formed. As he wandered the new universe his sweat became rivers, lakes, and the great oceans. His body hairs fell to become forests. Humans, taking not so illustrious a place, were the maggots that fell to earth from the giant's body.

A humble origin for humankind, this story contains elements that are important to understanding Chinese medical theory because it reveals the origin of *qì*. To abstract the terms of the myth to the contemporary parlance of Chinese medicine, yīn and yáng were separated from their primordial state, entering into a complex pattern of interrelated activities at the first moment of existence when Pán Gǔ cracked the cosmic egg.

This is expressed in an oft-encountered phrase among the classic writings on *tài jí quán*: "*Tài jí* comes from *wú jí* and is the mother of yīn and yáng." *Tài jí* means the "ultimate limit" or "boundaries of existence." *Wú jí* means "limitlessness" or "infinity." The existence of *qì* in the world, in the atmosphere, and in the channels and network vessels, is directly linked to the primordial differentiation of yīn and yáng. All of creation results from this cosmological evolution from limitlessness to the defining interrelationships of yīn and yáng. Among the great insights of the Daoist philosophers (which we will examine more closely in the following two chapters) is the recognition of *qì* as the third element of this cosmological formula. From the medical point of view, such insights have important implications.

We can begin to understand these implications when we ask doctors of traditional medicine what they are attempting to accomplish when administering treatment. We invariably learn that they are working to balance yīn and yáng, to harmonize the patient's *qì*. This doesn't mean that they want to return yīn and yáng to an original, undifferentiated state. It means that the dynamic balance of substance (yīn) and function (yáng) in the body has become disturbed, that it has gyrated beyond tolerable limits, and that the physician is endeavoring to set it right by applying the principles of yīn and yáng. Disease results from extremes, and a Chinese doctor's medical interventions, if only in some faint and imperceptible way, reflect the creation myth of Pán Gǔ.

Another important aspect of the Pán Gǔ story, from a medical point of view, is the creation of waterways and other geological features. The images of the myth are reflected in the conception of the *jīng luò* (channels and network vessels, or meridians) that course throughout the human body, communicating *qì* to every function and part. In fact, the mythic creation of earthly waterways and the waterway-like channels of *qì* are a mirror image of one another. In the myth, it is the weight of the giant's body that leaves impressions on the form of the earth. In *jīng luò* theory it is the *qì* coursing through its pathways in a symbolic, cyclic journey to the sea that determines the body's function and form.

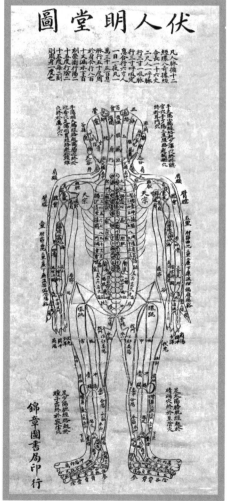

A 1914 chart showing posterior view of the circulation of qì through the jīng luò

In Chinese, the *jīng luò* and some acupoints that lie along them are described by analogy to flowing water. There are well, spring, stream, river, and sea points and many other points with names that associate aspects of the natural environment. This reflects the essential frame of reference for medical theorists in ancient China who viewed the human body as a microcosmic replica of the whole universe. The body is perceived as a system analogous to the world in which it lives. It has its valleys and ravines, hills, rivers, and windy places. It was also seen to have various structures that resembled in form and/or function elements of the human environment—granaries, storehouses, treasurehouses, marketplaces, cities, and streets.

We cannot hope to catalog herein all these names and the phenomena to which they refer. Our point is simply to demonstrate the Chinese conception of the structure and function of the body, of life itself, as

WHO CAN RIDE THE DRAGON?

an entirely integrated, comprehensive, and inclusive picture or pattern of pictures. By "picture," we mean an aesthetic perception, a comprehended image of the universe. The following quote from Sun Si Miao of the Tang Dynasty, one of China's most highly respected doctors, illustrates the pattern of images that filled the Chinese imagination.

> *Between heaven and earth, mankind is most precious.*
>
> *Man's head is round to symbolize the shape of heaven.*
>
> *The foot is square, symbolizing the earth.*
>
> *Heaven has four seasons; man has four limbs.*
>
> *Heaven has five phases; man has five viscera.*
>
> *Heaven has six extremes [i.e., upper, lower, north, south, east, and west]; man has six bowels.*
>
> *Heaven has eight winds [i.e., winds that blow from the eight cardinal points]; man has eight main joints.*
>
> *Heaven has nine stars; man has nine orifices.*
>
> *Heaven has twelve time periods; man has twelve channels.*
>
> *Heaven has twenty-four solar terms; man has twenty-four shù points [points running bilaterally along the spine that have particular effectiveness in mobilizing the qì of their corresponding internal organs].*
>
> *Heaven has three hundred and sixty five degrees; man has three hundred and sixty five bones and joints.*
>
> *Heaven has sun and moon; man has eyes.*
>
> *Heaven has day and night; man has wakening and sleep.*
>
> *Heaven has thunder and lightning; man has joy and anger.*
>
> *Heaven has rain and dew; man has snivel and tears.*
>
> *Heaven has yīn and yáng; man has cold and heat.*
>
> *Earth has springs and water; man has blood and vessels.*
>
> *Earth has grass and woods; man has hair on his skin and head.*
>
> *Earth has metal and stones; man has teeth.*

Our emphasis on this imagery is really no more than a way of underscoring the importance of a simple statement such as "Chinese medicine is holistic." Chinese medicine begins with a very basic supposition: human beings are microcosms of the whole universe. Thus we can see in the story of Pán Gǔ and the cosmic egg not just the birth of the universe, but the emergence of a set of universal images that weave through the vast Chinese cultural tapestry, animating the imaginations, language, theory, and ultimately the medical substances and practices of ancient and contemporary Chinese medicial doctors.

Foremost among these images are the images of *qì*. The transformation of original *qì* into the *qì* of heaven and earth is an essential concept underlying the entire theoretical infrastructure of Chinese medicine. In its primordial state, the existence of original *qì* meant that all things were One. The *qì* of yīn and yáng retains this connective or unifying potential. Chinese philosophers and medical theorists relied upon *qì* as the basis for explaining virtually all natural phenomena. They saw *qì* everywhere, from the movement of the stars to the food they ate.

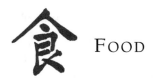 FOOD

If there is anything we're serious about, it is neither religion nor learning, but food.

LIN YU TANG

In our research of the topics covered in this book, we have spent a great deal of time simply listening to people. The stories, observations, philosophies, wisdom, emotions, and attitudes we have heard have become part of a constantly growing matrix of information by which we have developed understanding. One acquaintance tells the following story about Chinese attitudes towards food.

> *When I first came to China, I was working as an English teacher in local middle schools. My first big banquet was at the invitation of the head of the municipal education committee. He was a pleasant man in his 40's who spoke a little English. We sat beside each other as the food was served by lovely young women. Dish after more succulent dish of specialties I'd never dreamed of while eating in countless Chinese restaurants back in the States became the punctuation in our dinner conversation.*
>
> *Near the end of the meal, my host lifted his wine cup for what must have been the 20th time and offered me, in lieu of a toast, two pieces of advice that I've never forgotten.*
>
> *"First," he said lowering his cup so that he could speak to me over its lip, "be very careful when you are riding your bicycle."*

WHO CAN RIDE THE DRAGON?

I thanked him and was about to drink when he placed a finger lightly on my hand and bid me wait.

"Next," he continued with several knowing nods of his head, "if you want to understand us Chinese, pay attention to the way we eat!"

With that we emptied our wine cups and set at the platter most recently arrived. I think it was beef tendons swimming in a black bean sauce ... delicious.

There is another commonly heard story that underscores the importance of food in Chinese medicine. Many foreigners are surprised when offered a variety of Chinese dishes to learn the disease or medical condition that each plate of food can treat or ameliorate. "Everything they give me to eat is some sort of medicine!" exclaimed one expatriate executive after his first weeks in Hong Kong. The Chinese do indeed consider food not only as a satisfaction for hunger and as a delight for its delicious flavors but also as provision against human diseases. Food therapy is an ancient discipline in China, and Chinese quarters in cities around the world boast of marvelous eating establishments where medicinal fare is purveyed.

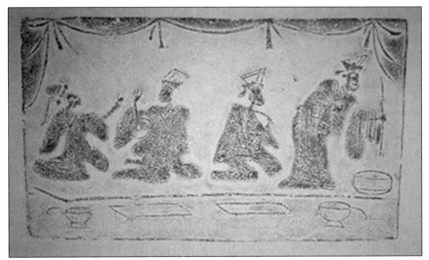

Stylized gestures reflecting the Chinese reverence for food are depicted in this rubbing of a Han Dynasty stone carving of a banquet

The link between food and herbs may seem obvious to some and obscure to others but in Chinese medicine there is a saying, "Medicine and food come from one source." Through their daily experiences with food, the ancient Chinese identified the flavors and natures of medicines as well as foods, categorizing them according to the same theories and observations. Mild-tasting plants were consumed regularly as food. Those with strong flavors and effects were considered medicines. Even the discovery of the most fundamental way of taking Chinese herbs—as a tea or soup—arose in ancient kitchens thousands of years ago. Herbs used every day in cooking—ginger, garlic, and onions, to name a few— are often found in medicinal formulas. Similarly, herbs treasured for their medicinal qualities are a common ingredient in Chinese dishes.

For example, chicken is often boiled in soup containing a ginseng or astragalus root, especially for elderly people who treasure these herbs as tonics for their *qì*. Many Chinese dishes contain the tiny red lycium berry, (*gǒu jǐ zǐ*) which is valued as an herb that supplements the yīn. These little red berries are frequently added to Chinese white wine, along with a wide array of other medicinals, making a glass of wine with a meal an integral part of a healthful dietary regimen.

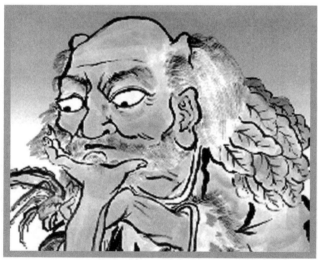

Shen Nong, from a painting by
Yoshio Manaka (circa 1984)

The traditional story of the invention of herbal medicine helps us understand the link between medicines and food. Shen Nong, one of the three original legendary emperors of China, who is said to have lived over 5000 years ago, is revered as the God of Agriculture. According to legend, he tasted hundreds of plants, discerning by flavor the nature of their *qì* and the medicinal properties they possessed.

WHO CAN RIDE THE DRAGON?

One glimpses in this simple ancient tale important kernels of understanding. The tradition of herbal medicine in China sprang from humankind's proximity with nature in the ancient world, developing through a long process of trial and error and evolving as an integral aspect of the natural consumption of agricultural products.

This is a widespread phenomenon. Peoples everywhere have developed their understanding of the medicinal properties of the plants that grow in their native regions. In the traditions of Chinese medicine we have access to thousands of years of practical development and refinement of practical experience, and it has been only recently that modern Western societies have temporarily lost this knowledge. Today in many Western societies, there is a widespread reemergence of interest in, and understanding of, the relationship between plants, herbs, food, human nutrition, medicine, and wellbeing. It is this awareness that the Chinese have cultivated and refined for thousands of years.

Beginning in the Zhou Dynasty (1066–770 B.C.E.), the position of Imperial Dietician or *Shí Yī* was created. From that time forward, there was always a *shí yī* in the emperor's court. The work of these dieticians had a strong, positive effect on the widespread use of medicinal herbs. During the period of the Warring States (475–221 B.C.E.), the famous doctor Bian Que stated:

> *To be a doctor one must understand the origin of disease clearly. [One must] know which part of the body has been invaded and treat it with food. If diet cannot cure the disease, then prescribe the medicinal formula.*

Even the most revered book of Chinese medicine, the *Yellow Emperor's Canon of Internal Medicine,* advises, "Use medicinal herbs to eliminate illness and follow the formula with a diet that will nourish the patient." In these examples we see clearly how diet and medicine were understood as a single approach to illness that extended beyond the acute stage of disease to provide nourishment for recovery. Through the 3000 years of diet therapy in China there have been many books in each dynasty devoted to the subject. These serve as a guide for those who seek to control and harmonize their instinctual hunger for food. Indeed, the urge to eat is one of the most basic urges, and Chinese dietary traditions provide us with an invaluable knowledge and wisdom about the qualities and functions of specific foods. Long before there were theories or techniques for manufacturing medicine, people relied upon this knowledge to guide their eating and to treat their symptoms.

Of course, this knowledge developed from the same notion of *qì* that we see in the myth of Pán Gǔ, the *qì* that escaped from the cosmic egg, the *qì* that nourishes all creation. Thus, the relationship between people and the food they ate was described in terms of *qì*. Food plants and herbs were categorized according to their flavors and their *qì*. This ancient rudimentary system of classifying herbs survives to the present in the basis of Chinese herbal medicine.

 ## Marriage and Family Obligations

In traditional Chinese life, there is no occasion more solemn than marriage. As in feudal societies everywhere, marriage was a social and political institution that consolidated power and relationships between families, states, and nations. Yet even when no such grand design is involved, marriage in China is approached in the most serious manner.

Traditionally, marriages were arranged by the parents of the bride and groom, sometimes years in advance. These arrangements were typically concluded without consideration for the couple's feelings because marriage, both in ritual and reality, served not solely to establish a new family unit but also to provide the basic pattern for development of family and social life. These issues were far more important than mere emotions. By arranging suitable marriages for their children, parents ensured their own futures as well as those of their children. As such, it was regarded as an inviolable social institution created by no less a figure than Fu Xi, another of the three legendary emperors of China's prehistory.

The limits of marriage were not, however, as strictly defined as they are in modern Western cultures, which see monogamy as the central theme of marriage. In traditional China, the number of women with whom a man could associate was determined by his financial capability, not by the tenets of philosophy or religion. The social custom was for a wealthy man to have a wife and many concubines. Those who were poorer could afford a few or only one.

Among the many women in wealthy households there was a hierarchical order that reflected the Confucian sense of duty and responsibility. The specific list of duties and responsibilities, although not endless, was onerously long. It included matters such as the positions at which one could sit for meals, the rights and privileges of offspring, access to and influence over the male head of the household. It should be noted though that like social strictures everywhere, such rules were frequently bent or broken but never discarded.

It is a curious fact of contemporary China that such multiple "marriages" (which are no longer officially recognized), are once again gaining popularity as more Chinese men acquire the financial resources required to support several wives. In a 1995 radio broadcast, the Mayor of Shen Zhen, the economic boomtown across from what was once the border between Hong Kong and China, described the keeping of many wives as the number-one social problem facing his city. Shen Zhen is the city annointed by no less a person than the late Deng Xiao Ping as the model for future growth and development in China. In China today, to be rich is not only glorious, but also an opportunity to reestablish traditional values.

It was this set of values, rooted firmly in the institution of marriage, that provided Chinese people with stability in their day-to-day lives. Wives had their subset of values, duties, and responsibilities. Husbands had theirs. Responsibility was not limited to these two positions in the family. Well-defined patterns of responsibility and privilege extended to every member of a family. This reflects a principle from the Confucian classic, *Zhōng Yōng (The Unwobbling Pivot)*, as translated by Ezra Pound.

> *The man of breeding looks at his own status, seeing it in a clear light without trimmings; he acts, and lusts not after things extraneous to it. Finding himself rich and honored he behaves as befitting one who is rich and honored; finding himself of low estate he behaves as is fitting for a man of low estate.*

The same can be understood to apply to each and every member of a Chinese family; each occupies their own distinct position within the microcosmic structure of their own family and the macrocosm of society itself.

This same concern for the traditional concept of the proper arrangement of things manifested in medical theory in the "social organization" of the body. The internal organs are understood to be the rulers, ministers, and officals of bodily affairs. They communicate, exchange, and in the case of illness, contest with one another through the medium of the body's *qì*, the *qì* that escaped from Pán Gǔ's egg. Qì flows incessantly between yīn and yáng throughout the natural environment, the Great *Qì* of heaven and earth organizes the entirety of the human being as a functional unit according to the hierarchical structure of both the Chinese family and Chinese society in general.

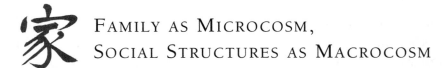 FAMILY AS MICROCOSM, SOCIAL STRUCTURES AS MACROCOSM

One humane family can humanize the whole state. One courteous family can lift a whole state into courtesy. One grasping and perverse man can drive a nation to chaos.

These words from Ezra Pound's translation of the Confucian classic *Dà Xué (The Great Learning)* describe a deeply held belief in traditional Chinese culture. If it can generally be said that the family forms the basic organizing unit or principle of human society, then China is an outstanding example of this universal characteristic. The family has played a central role in the lives of Chinese people for so long that many in China today feel strongly that this societal foundation is invulnerable to the social forces running virtually wild in China's rapid expansion.

When we suggest to Chinese colleagues that the same social stresses and strains that have so heavily undermined the American family in the past several decades could have a similar effect on the character, if not the structure, of the family in China, the usual response is the self-assured assumption that "the family is too important in Chinese life . . . too ancient . . . too well established" to give way to television, the internet, drugs, or teenage violence. Despite statistics that show a sharp increase in divorce and a general deterioration of family values and traditional roles during the past ten to fifteen years, many Chinese continue to think of the family as the unfailing heart beating at the center of their civilization.

This reliance upon the immutable image of the family and the importance of filial relationships is, of course, evident in Chinese medicine. Familial relationships are used as metaphors expressing the patterns of relationships between the internal organs and the transformations of *qì* that occur in physiology and pathology. Chinese medical doctors speak, for example, of the "mother" organ providing birth and nourishment to the "son" as a way of explaining the pattern of *qì* generation within the body. This pattern of interrelationships is based on the theory of the five phases and is used to predict and prevent the progression of disease. These images are pervasive thoughout Chinese medicial theory, just as familial relationships remain powerful and persistent images filling the minds and hearts of Chinese people wherever they live.

The blueprint for the Chinese family, and the social organization of the body that Chinese medicine describes, are to a large extent founded on the writings of Confucius. These set forth the position of a man and his family based on the four most basic relationships: *jūn chén fù zǐ*. This means, "king, minister, father, and son." These are the essential elements of patriarchy and are thought to reflect universal order. These positions are delineated as rights, duties, and responsibilities within the familial and social hierarchies, as well as in the principles of Chinese medicine where these relationships describe the interactions of constituents in medicinal formulas. [See Chapters 3 and 4 for more detailed discussions of the Confucian "blueprint" of social order and its relationship to medicine.]

What we see reflected in the Confucian ideals of the family, as in the past and present lives of the Chinese people, is a set of values, beliefs, and attitudes that have evolved though thousands of years. One of the key elements supporting this value system is its significance to duration or longevity. There is an important Chinese word that expresses this essential value and it provides the keystone of a bridge of understanding between Chinese and Western cultures. That word is *cháng* 长. In literal translation this character means "long." The same character, pronounced *zhǎng,* means "to grow." But its meaning runs deep below these literal surfaces.

In Chinese the Great Wall is *Cháng Chéng,* or "long wall." Clearly a connotation other than mere length is intended and understood when the Chinese use this word to describe one of the most important monuments of their civilization. This character is also used in another expression of enormous importance in China: *cháng shòu,* "long life." *Cháng shòu* is not merely a long span of years, it is a blessing of heaven. It is the great reward to be reaped by properly following the various formulas and principles that have developed through centuries of experimentation aimed at lengthening life and maintaining youth. This fundamental value, this overriding concern for longevity and duration, has informed medical practice since ancient times.

That which is long, to Chinese eyes, has value, has root. That which is not long is gone. The Chinese place a profound importance on age, the accumulation of experience, knowledge, and understanding that can gradually develop to wisdom. Thus, we can understand why elders have a special place and a particular import in the Chinese family. Just as Americans sometimes lie about their age to appear younger, Chinese will add a year or two to make the cloak of their lives appear more elaborate, more impressive. We knew one old gentleman, a doctor and teacher of *tài jí quán* who, in the several months of our close association, aged nearly eight years!

Similarly, the age of the family itself is enormously important in the traditional perspective. For example, it is a common boast of doctors of Chinese medicine that they come from a lineage that is comprised of several, if not dozens or more, generations of doctors. Where this seems mildly interesting or perhaps even impressive to a Westerner, in those cases where it is true, it is a mark of rare distinction for a Chinese. Not only is the presence of family secrets thereby suggested, but those with a multigenerational lineage are thought to possess something by birthright that others lack.

This concern is not limited to medical families. Virtually every family with sufficient means keeps a family book or annal in which the names, births, weddings, deaths, and vital facts of all its members are recorded. A curious feature and function of these annals is the naming of generations. Names are given to each generation so that every member of that generation has one name in common with every brother, sister, and cousin born in their generation. One reason and result of this custom in traditional China was the ability to know simply when hearing someone's name where they fit in a family's generational hierarchy. Again, this reflects the importance of one's sense of place in the established order. Knowing this, individuals were connected to something much grander than themselves.

This same sensibility can be seen at work in the traditional concept of the body as a family made of the internal organs. Each organ had its proper "place" and function in Chinese medical theory. If the organs all behaved accordingly, then the whole body enjoyed wholeness and harmony. It was therefore easy to understand and express the physiological disturbances of disease in metaphorical terms using these relations. The Chinese medical phrase, *zǐ dào mǔ qì*, for example, means literally "the son steals the mother's *qì*." This phrase is applied to a common pathological condition affecting the heart and liver. According to the theory of the five phases, the liver, which is associated with the wood phase, is the mother of the heart, which is associated with the fire phase. In other words, the fire of the heart is born of the liver. But if the heart fire is replete, so hot and active that it exceeds its accustomed bounds, it will consume the yīn of the liver. The son—the heart—steals the yīn of the mother—the liver. The family metaphor thus conveys not only a specific understanding of pathology but a qualitative image of disharmony that is not only rooted in the idea of orginal *qì*, but supported by all the cultural influences expressed in the myth of Pán Gǔ.

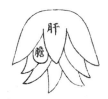

early woodcut depicting the liver (gān zàng)

The whole point of this yearning for harmony is to establish the basis of longevity, as expressed in the Chinese character *cháng,* mentioned above. The longevity of the family, as in the West, was understood to be transmitted from father to son, the male aspect of the generational synapse. Traditionally, the leadership of a family is bestowed on the father. The organizing principle resides in the mother. This reflects the notion of yīn (female and nutritive) and yáng (male and active) applied to human relationships. For countless generations it has provided the essential structural integrity of family life, hence social life, in China.

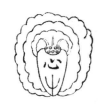

early woodcut depicting the heart (xīn zàng)

Whenever yīn and yáng are present, there is *qì*. The harmonious interaction of father and mother, of parents and children, as well as all familial relationships, establishes the basis for the necessary transformations that accompany successive generations as the family flourishes and develops. In other words, the balance of yīn and yáng within the family results in the *qì* of the family flowing smoothly on, as seen in the Chinese ideal of "four generations under one roof."

This has been reflected in the basic societal structures of imperial China since the first Emperor. Another traditional name for the leader of China is "The Son of Heaven."

Heaven symbolizes pure yáng, the male element. The mantle of leadership passes to Earth from Heaven via the Emperor who is thereby the father of the nation. This lineage extends throughout the complex bureaucratic structure of the government and distributes political and economic power throughout the country. The influence of this system reflects the family and stands as a microcosm of society and the universe itself.

These ideas and images were incorporated directly, if metaphorically, into the theories and terms of Chinese medicine. The principle of "governance" is an example of a typical medical metaphor. The channel that runs along the spine from the perineum to the headtop is known as the *dū mài* or Governing Vessel. It is understood to be the most yáng of the yáng channels, and thus the movement of *qì* in the *dū mài* governs the movement of *yáng qì* throughout the body.

This concept mirrors the design by ancient architects of the social contract in China. The quote from the Confucian classic, the *Dà Xué* (see p. 56), illustrates this point precisely. The Chinese have long held in common the view that for the country to flourish, family life must be maintained in good order. Thus relationships between family members acquired enormous importance, subtle meanings, and specific characteristics. One's place in the family, to a great extent, determined how one's life would develop and unfold.

Chinese medicine is profoundly influenced by this aspect of the social milieu in which it has developed. The whole sense of organization of the structures and functions of the body reflects the same characteristic Chinese predilection for order and harmony that are apparent in the ideals of family life and its corresponding social structures. Thus, within the theoretical framework of Chinese medicine, the internal organs themselves operate like a family, each with its relative importance and particular role to play.

Those who are familiar with Chinese traditional diagnostic methods, as well as with the principles of formulating treatment plans and acupoint prescriptions in the clinical application of acupuncture, are no doubt familiar with the mother–son relationship mentioned above. The images of mother and son are not merely poetic metaphors, because they also succinctly encode the therapeutic relationships that the ancient Chinese masters of medicine discovered. They are precise observations that reflect a clear, comprehensive understanding of how the whole body is integrated into a functional whole. It, like other medical metaphors and literary devices, is a tool that when properly understood and applied, guides practitioners to effective methods for diagnosing and treating disease.

More importantly, these theories can guide us to a sense of the harmony of the body/mind/spirit that is envisioned and made attainable through the theories and methods of Chinese medicine. These theories reflect the generally held view in Chinese thought that the universe is a series of micro- and macrocosmic interrelationships established between the three principal realms—heaven, earth, and humankind. Harmony of body and mind, as harmony in heaven and earth, can only be achieved through harmonizing the *qì*. Not only does such a view provide Chinese people with medical theories and practices, it serves to connect them with their ancient past.

 # CONTINUITY FROM ANCIENT TIMES TO THE PRESENT

One important aspect of the Chinese collective experience and worldview is the continuity of what it means to be Chinese. Where it may be difficult for the people of any nationality to consider that their nation might disappear, for the Chinese it is virtually impossible.

This is not to suggest that Chinese cannot conceive of and execute revolutionary change in their intra- and international relations. The history of the 20th century proves the Chinese capable of extraordinary and revolutionary change. Neither do the Chinese have a merely geographic image of themselves. Indeed, as an old saying in China goes, "Sometimes we're together and sometimes we're apart." It is used to describe the historic ebb and flow of relations between various regions and provinces.

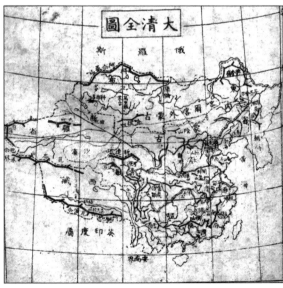

Map of the Qing Empire

Folk Beliefs, Myths, and Customs

Yet, through the rising and receding tides of history, China continues, perhaps more a state of mind than a nation state. This continuity provides the Chinese people, and therefore Chinese culture and its various manifestations, a characteristic sense of self that is reflected in its cultural, scientific, intellectual, and artistic achievements. This "sense of themselves" is characterized by several important attributes.

First, there is a sense of permanence. To be Chinese is to be a part of something that has withstood the test of time. We might say that those artifacts the Chinese have found indispensable have been subjected to centuries of trial and error. Through natural selection, the Chinese people have proven their traditional ways of thinking and their traditional methods for solving fundamental existential problems. Thus, they have established to their own satisfaction that they are competent, qualified, and can be depended on to persist. From any objective view of history, this is difficult to dispute.

The reemergence of the traditional trend towards multiple marriages is just one of many reemerging traditional values and customs. Contemporary Chinese enthusiastically accept Western advancements in science and technology, and they are anxious to surpass their Western colleagues. Nonetheless, the Chinese continue to embrace many of their ancient views and traditions. The most ancient of these views is that the essence of life is change.

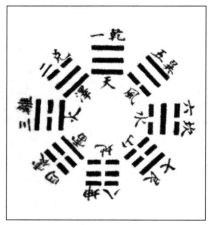

Bà Guà—the eight basic images of the Yì Jīng

If there is a single traditional wisdom that has enabled the Chinese to preserve and refine their cultural identity, it is the notion of change. It is no coincidence that the oldest, most respected (even if not the most understood) of the Chinese classics is the *Classic of Change,* the Yì Jīng. (See Chapter 4 for a more detailed discussion of the Yì Jīng.). The Chinese fashioned a cultural method for deriving a sense of permanence from its apparent opposite—change—and ironically, the complex variations of Chinese history emerge as the essence of its continuity.

This subtle and intricate concept of permanence through change is of enormous importance in medical theory and practice. A well-trained

WHO CAN RIDE THE DRAGON?

doctor of Chinese medicine does not see patients as static images or snapshots. Patients' symptoms and signs are understood in a comprehensive theory of diagnosis based on recognizing dynamic patterns of disease. These pathological patterns are always in a state of change. Medical interventions are thus understood to be coordinated interactions meant to shift the disease process away from deeper and more serious progression. This permits a doctor of Chinese medicine to treat patients before they become *more* ill, that is, to ameliorate the course of a disease before it becomes untreatable. This prognostic aspect of Chinese medicine is one of its most attractive characteristics, but one possible only for those who understand how the ancient medical theorists perceived and analyzed their world.

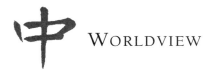 WORLDVIEW

The question, "What is the Chinese worldview?" is not easily answered. When considering the vast range of topics that could be discussed, one idea leaps to prominence. We call this salient point "centrality" because the Chinese word, *zhōng,* center, is enormously important in Chinese life. Like so many Chinese words it has many meanings and even more connotations, attitudes, and associated feelings.

First and foremost, it means "center," "middle." In the character, 中 we see a simple schematic of a center; the relationship of the elements graphically indicate the meaning. This character derives from the ancient pictograph for a flagpole. It is a term that appears in numerous important concepts. First, it is the name of China, which in Chinese has nothing to do with the Qin ("Chin") Dynasty from which our English word is derived. The Chinese call their homeland "The Central Country" or "The Middle Kingdom."

It is common for nations to consider themselves the center of the world. Maps published in the United States place the USA at the center of the world. For an American schoolchild, the United States *is* the center of the world, enforcing the natural impressions one's homeland encourages. This is also true for Chinese schoolchildren. The United States in not the center of the maps on their classroom walls. It is China, the Central Country, that occupies that place. An American seeing these maps for the first time must repress the urge to blurt out, "Hey, your map is all wrong. The USA should be in the center."

To develop an understanding of traditional Chinese culture, Chinese medicine, and related subjects, it is necessary to understand what the Chinese mean when they say Zhōng Guó, the "Central Kingdom." Over the millennia of Chinese history the instinct to perceive and behave in self-centered ways has developed into a highly complex view of the world in which the Chinese see themselves and their culture as central, not just in Asia, but in all the world. Throughout history the Chinese people have seen other kingdoms rise and fall. The borders of China have vacillated, making Chinese territory larger, then smaller, then larger again. At times, foreign hordes swept across the frontiers, establishing hegemony and controlling the capital. Yet China endured. Age after age, dynasty after dynasty, invasion after invasion, the Central Kingdom moved through human history, as if other states and kingdoms revolved around it.

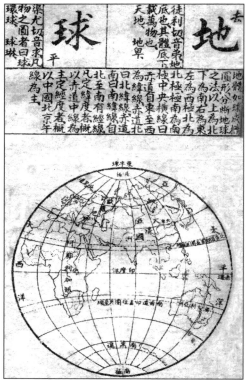

Chinese world map from a Qing Dynasty illustrated dictionary

The Chinese have also been seafaring for centuries. Long before Europeans ventured onto the high seas, when the West was still befuddled by the Church's unworkable flat-earth dogma, Chinese traders sailed throughout Southeast Asia, India, Africa, Central Asia and the Middle East. In what we call the "Middle Ages," long before international conventions or intellectual property rights, the Chinese freely shared their fundamental discoveries in science and technology, providing some of the intellectual spark for the Western renaissance. China and the Chinese people have not only been a well of innovation, they have also been the source of technologies with which to survive and prosper. Thus, they view themselves as central in world affairs.

WHO CAN RIDE THE DRAGON?

Chinese medical knowledge is far from the least of China's intellectual contributions to the family of man, and although most Chinese share the view that the importance and power of the Central Kingdom has ebbed in recent centuries, it too evidences this spirit of survival. Neglected, ignored, and outlawed at the end of the 19th and beginning of the 20th centuries, China's native medical traditions have once again resurrected. In the caves of Yan An, Mao Ze Dong and his followers relied on whatever medical means they could acquire. The economy and efficacy of acupuncture and Chinese medicine were indispensable to the guerilla army that ultimately conquered and once again unified China in 1949. Ever since, the Chinese government has steadily fostered the growth and development of a "world medicine" movement aimed at integrating traditional medicine with modern healthcare delivery.

In December of 1997, the State Administration of Traditional Chinese Medicine in Beijing adopted a 10-year plan to promote the dissemination and integration of Traditional Chinese Medicine (T.C.M.) around the world. Given the rapid increase in doctors and patients turning to Chinese medicine worldwide, this program seems destined to succeed, bringing into clear focus an important dimension of the traditional Chinese worldview.

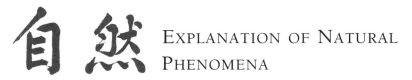 EXPLANATION OF NATURAL PHENOMENA

One of the lessons we learned from studying Chinese language and literature is that the form of a work must correspond to its contents. If this were a book of folktales, this section would be different. However, since the vital connections between Chinese medicine and its cultural background are fundamental ingredients in traditional Chinese stories, myths, and tales, traditional Chinese explanations for the origins of all things occupy our focus.

In contrast to modern physics, which has been almost exclusively concerned with the essential building blocks of the physical world, the ancient Chinese developed rich expressions for nature and natural phenomena based on the concept of transforming qi. It is therefore of primary importance that we come to terms with this idea if we are to grasp the meaning of Chinese medical theories and techniques. It is hard to imagine a modern heart surgeon performing a delicate bypass of the coronary arteries without a comprehensive description of the heart, the body it animates, and to some extent the world in which that body lives and to which its heart responds. It is equally difficult to conceive of using an acupuncture needle without knowing where to put it, what to do with it, and why, without understanding how the Chinese thought of *qì*. That knowledge can only come from understanding the traditional Chinese schematic of the body and the environmental matrix that creates and supports its growth and development.

All traditional Chinese explanations begin with *qì*. However, to deal with the complex manifestations of *qì*, ancient philosophers, cosmologists, and medical theorists described the three elemental treasures with which humankind is gifted: *jīng*, *qì*, and *shén*. All the substances that exist within the body are understood as manifestations of these three treasures. As the body itself is understood to be a microcosm of the universe, for the ancient Chinese, the whole universe consisted of *jīng*, *qì*, and *shén*.

jīng

After yīn and yáng, the three treasures can be understood as the next stratum of complexity in the taxonomic organization of phenomena in Chinese philosophical and medical traditions. Among those who follow such traditions, *jīng*, *qì*, and *shén* are virtually always described as the three treasures of the body. But, what is *jīng*? What is *qì*? What is *shén*? The answers depend on understanding *qì*.

qì

The problem of how to translate the Chinese word *qì* is complex. It is clear that Chinese philosophers held that *qì*, specifically original *qì*, was responsible for the creation of the universe, and that once created, the universe was bound together by *qì*. In the Spring and Autumn Period (770–475 B.C.E.) Zhuang Zi, one of the

shén

WHO CAN RIDE THE DRAGON?

legendary founders of Daoism, stated this clearly: "Throughout all creation, there is only one *qì*." By then, the ancient Chinese had already described how heaven, earth, water, fire, the moon, and the sun were created. In terms that echo the myth of Pán Gǔ, *Qián Záo Dù* (*The Classic of Astronomy*) says:

> There was only an enshrouding mist before heaven and earth came into existence. This is called the Great Beginning. The Great Beginning gave birth to the Shape of the Void. The Shape of the Void gave birth to the Universe. The Universe gave birth to *qì*.
>
> Thus the *qì* is limited. The light [aspect of the] *qì* rises to become heaven. The heavy [aspect of the] *qì* sinks and congeals to become earth. The light and fine [aspect of] *qì* is simpler than the murky *qì*. Thus heaven came before earth.

In a later passage of this book it is written:

> The *qì* of heat comes from the accumulation of *yáng* and gives birth to fire. The essence [*jīng*] of the *qì* of fire is the sun.
>
> The cold *qì* comes from the accumulation of *yīn* and gives birth to water. The essence of the *qì* of water is the moon.

In short, everything on earth and in heaven is created from *qì* and the qualities of *qì* as described by *yīn* and *yáng* are rigorously expressed in all creation.

Ancient Chinese philosophers proposed that "When the *qì* of heaven and earth interact, everything is given birth." The *Yellow Emperor's Canon of Internal Medicine* (*Sù Wèn*) says:

> In heaven it is *qì* [mist]. On earth it takes shape. When *qì* and shape engage in intercourse, they give birth to everything on earth.

The Chinese consider that *qì* is something too insubstantial to perceive. It unfolds into the vast atmosphere in which all things exist. Yet it is constantly moving and changing and by understanding the changes of observable phenomena we can become aware of *qì*. Creation owes its existence to the transformations of *qì*. Creation is the movement of *qì*. Were this movement to stop, there would be no change in the universe—there would be no universe. Naturally then, *qì* creates the whole world and every part of the world is full of *qì*. It fills the space between all shapes, all objects. It fills the void between heaven and earth. It fills the gaps that separate things and connects them. It exists among people,

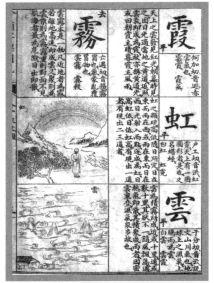

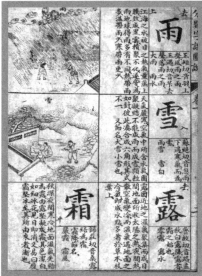

Illustrations from a late Qing Dynasty encyclopedic dictionary describe various atmospheric phenomena such as rain, snow, dew, clouds, rainbows, fog, and dusk. All are understood as manifestations of "yún qì" or the qì of the clouds, as can be seen in the following excerpts:

"Rain: the waters of rivers and the sea are vaporized by the warm qì and gather to form black clouds that produce the rain."

"Snow: when the weather is cold, the watery qì in the air cannot sustain itself and becomes frozen turning to snow and frost."

and between people and nature. *Qì* is the medium of existence, connecting everything in the universe, making it whole, unified.

That human beings are a part of this wholeness is the fundamental assertion of Chinese philosophy, Chinese medical theory, and the traditional Chinese view of life. Of particular importance to medical theory is the belief that *qì* creates human life. "The Treatise on the Complete Treasure of Life" in the *Sù Wèn* section of the *Yellow Emperor's Canon of Internal Medicine* says, "Human beings are created by the *qì* of heaven and earth. Their growth follows the pattern of the four seasons." A later quotation from the same work says, "Of the intercourse between heaven and earth, their *qì* creates humankind."

The material substance which comprises the human body is, in these terms, the combined *qì* of heaven and earth. Here we see again the gist of the tale of Pán Gǔ reflected in a medical theory. The dynamic potential of yīn and yáng, established by cracking the cosmic egg, gives rise to the vital processes that form and animate the human body. This *qì* is the transformative potential that impels the forces we know as human life. Moreover, the flow of *qì* throughout the body binds it into a living organism. The internal organs, the blood, the whole body, and its external movements all depend on *qì* for the impetus to function.

WHO CAN RIDE THE DRAGON?

Thus when the *qì* is dense and vibrant, the person will be healthy and full of vitality. When the *qì* is sparse and weak, the person will be sick or impaired. When the *qì* moves in an unnatural or abnormal direction, or when it moves when it should be still, illness will arise. *Qì* not only creates life; it sustains life and gives it quality. An ancient saying from the *Yellow Emperor's Canon of Internal Medicine* expresses this idea: "When the *qì* gathers, it takes shape. When the *qì* is lost, this shape disappears."

Given the context of *qì*, what is meant by the Chinese word *jīng?* In Chinese medicine, there are different concepts contained within the word: "refined, essence, extraction, perfect, excellent, meticulous, fine, smart, sharp, skilled, proficient, energy, spirit, sperm, seed, semen, extremely, goblin, spirit, demon, the fundamental substance which maintains the functionality of the body, the essence of life." It is used in reference to the refined part of all the *qì* in the universe, all the useful entities within the human body, and the essence stored within the kidneys.

jīng

The concept of *jīng* is metaphorically encapsulated in the character itself. This character consists of two elements. On the left is the character *mǐ*, which means "rice" or "grain." The right side is the character *qīng*, which means "green" and "youth." In the Ming Dynasty, a doctor named Xu Jun explained the meaning of *jīng* by saying that the combination of *mǐ* and *qīng* yields *jīng*. To understand this image, we must consider the significance of rice in Chinese life, where it has long been the staple grain. For countless generations of Chinese, the appearance of the young green rice sprouts symbolizes the regeneration of life itself.

mǐ

Were it not for the seasonal emergence of this phenomenon of the green rice sprouts, life would cease. Xu Jun evokes and illuminates this powerful symbol of the essence of life in his explanation that "the young green rice means essence." In this potent self-contained metaphor we also see the implicit significance of the generative principle of *jīng,* just as the farmer beheld the renewal of life in the springtime sprouting of his rice

qīng

Folk Beliefs, Myths, and Customs

crop. In medicine, *qīng* is the color associated with spring and the phase of wood, growth, and the renewal of life after its retreat to the seed state in winter.

In Chinese medical texts, as well as in daily parlance among Chinese practitioners of traditional medicine, the term *jīng qì* is common. This compounded use reflects the understanding that *jīng* is a manifestation of and can only function in relation to *qì*. This basic theoretical precept was probably in some part adapted from the philosophy of Guan Zi who lived and wrote in the Warring States period (475–221 B.C.E.). He used the word *jīng qì* to discuss *qì*. His work marks a major development in the study of *qì* as philosophy in China. This philosophical influence on Chinese medical theory manifests in an understanding of the cyclical transformations of life. Chinese medical theory holds that the *jīng qì* is the essence from which the human body is created. *Jīng qì* is not merely the reproductive essence, the semen or egg. Nor is it solely any particular aspect of the universe or human body, it is the essence of life itself.

Jīng exists implicitly before birth in the cycle of human creation. It is formed at the moment of conception from the merging of the *jīng qì* of the parents. It is this fundamental *jīng qì* that becomes the substantial basis of the new life thus created, its growth and, eventually, reproduction. When the *jīng qì* enters (creates) a body, that body is endowed with a reserve of this essence of life. Only then is the body quickened to support and sustain life and growth.

It would not be possible to practice Chinese medicine without a comprehensive and authentic understanding of *jīng*. Chinese medical theorists hold that virtually every phenomenon related to the human body is a manifestation of the dynamic potentials contained within the essence of life, the *jīng qì*.

What then, is *shén*? The word has four basic meanings: 1. The implicit law and expression of the movements and transformations of substances in the natural world; 2. The master (governing principle) of people's lives; 3. The exterior manifestation of life; 4. The human mind; consciousness, spirit. In the *Sù Wèn* it states:

> *The birth of life is called transformation. The extreme of substances is known as change. The immeasurable movements of yīn and yáng are called shén.*

WHO CAN RIDE THE DRAGON?

In the *Xìng Mìng Guī Zhǐ* it says:

> *It gives birth to life. You can see it nourish life only in life's growth. It brings life to its end. You can see it damage life only in life's disappearance. It is called shén.*

Shén is the least substantial of the three treasures because it is the spirit, the spark of heaven that provides the vitality of life to the living. In traditional China the spiritual dimension of existence was complex. The notion of an eternal or heavenly spirit that dwells within the human breast is contained in the word *shēn*. It is associated with the heart, the monarch of the internal organs. The heart is also understood to be the seat of consciousness. Thus the readers of Chinese works in translation are occasionally confused because the Chinese word *xīn*, heart, means both "heart" and "mind." In traditional Chinese physiology, control of mental processes including consciousness, thinking, and the emotions, belong to the various functions of the heart.

shén

This reflects an ancient belief, in no way unique to China, that the human mind is a reflection of divine intelligence. The concept of *shén* as the link between heaven and humankind is contained in the pictographic roots of the word. *Shén* has two components. The right side of the character is the radical *shēn*. It lends its sound to the character. In addition, it lends its meaning as the ninth of the ten heavenly stems, divisions of time in a complex system for measuring and dividing days, months, and years according to the ancient Chinese lunar calendar. The period of the day corresponding with *shēn* was the time when the Zhou emperor's counselors would gather to hear and discuss his edicts. The emperor's position as "the son of heaven" thus reflects the link between the divine and the human that is implicit in the word *shén*. For on the left side of *shén* we find the character shì 示 which is depicted as 礻 when it appears as an element of a compound character. It is a pictograph described in the *Shuō Wén Jiě Zì*, China's oldest extant dictionary, as follows:

Folk Beliefs, Myths, and Customs

Shì is heaven handing down a manifestation to instruct mankind concerning good and bad fortune. Its meaning follows from èr [the character "two," present in shì as the upper two lines and here is a reference to the "two-ness" of yīn and yáng]. The three manifestations [represented by the lower three lines] are the sun, the moon, and the stars. To observe the heavenly language, to inspect the changes of the seasons, shì instructs the will of God.

Thus the complete meaning of *shén* begins to emerge. Not only does the word mean "spirit," in the sense described above, it also has the meaning of "God." The presence of *shén* in the human body thus clearly expresses the eternal spark of divine mystery and intelligence that links humans to heaven and provide divine guidance through the mysterious transformations of life.

The *Sù Wèn* says, "If one has *shén* he is full of life. But if he loses his *shén*, he will die." This meaning of *shén* is typically expressed in the word *shén qì*, just as we saw with *jīng*. When a Chinese doctor prepares to examine a patient, the doctor needs to know the state of the patient's *shén qì*. In technical terms, how is their spiritedness? Is their tone and voice rich? Is their bearing upright? Is their conception and expression clear and responsive? These are the primary determining observations in prognosis, based upon the above-cited principle from the *Sù Wèn*.

The last three of the above meanings are particularly important within the context of Chinese medicine. The word also means "god, divinity, supernatural, magical, mind, expression, look, smart, clever." Throughout history, medical doctors, philosophers (especially Daoists), and all who sought to preserve their health understood and appreciated these three treasures, *jīng*, *qì*, and *shén*. They understood that health of body and mind, and therefore life itself, depended on treasuring these gifts. If someone lacked of any one of these three treasures, they could not preserve life or health.

Jīng, *qì*, and *shén* provided ancient theorists with an irreducible minimum description of the matrix that was the foundation of life and all its expressions. The search for unity, and its development in human life, has been a fundamental aim of Chinese medicine for centuries and it is with these concepts that they addressed the mysteries of life and death.

WHO CAN RIDE THE DRAGON?

生死 LIFE AND DEATH

If you walk down the streets of a Chinese city, sooner or later you will encounter a curious site. Large wreaths constructed of many-colored paper will stand three, four, or more deep at the entrance of a family home. Outside, inside, everywhere you look as you pass by, you will see tables full of *majiang (mah-jongg)* players, card players, and the like. Always, if you look carefully towards the back of the front room, you will find a somber black and white photograph of someone, usually old, with a stern expression.

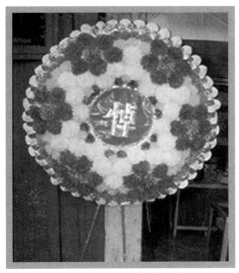

A funeral wreath with the Chinese character for "grief"

The tables are strewn with fruit and snacks. Wine and beer flow in and out of glasses. The guests at this gathering sometimes emerge and look around the street with lost, empty eyes as if searching for someone who isn't there. Pass by the same house on consecutive days and you find this party continues steadily for three days and three nights, the established period for the celebration of "the white," the passing of the dead.

Celebrations of "the red" and "the white" are the most important affairs in China. These are the colors of death (white) and marriage (red). Earlier in Chapter 2, we presented a discussion of the celebrations of red. Here, we focus on traditional Chinese attitudes, beliefs, and customs concerning two equally important issues: life and death.

One day while working in the clinic at the hospital at the Chengdu University of Traditional Chinese Medicine, we asked the Director of the acupuncture department what had happened to a patient whose case we had been following.

"He has no *qì*," answered Dr. Wang, looking down at his desk. "What do you mean?" "Aiyah!" replied Dr. Wang, tapping his finger on his desk and wrinkling his brow as he did when we failed to grasp the obvious. "He died."

The next day, members of the man's family came to the clinic to invite the doctor to the funeral, and we accompanied him to pay our respects to the family and to the man whose life could not be saved. It was a scene very much like the one described above. Not without grieving and certainly not a celebration, this Chinese funeral was an observance of a natural phenomenon. We were curious to know Dr. Wang's thoughts about the loss of his patient. His laconic expression said little, yet answered everything. "Yīn and yáng separated. That means life is at its end. Nothing to be done."

For Westerners, it can be hard to understand Chinese attitudes toward religion and faith. A central issue in most religions is the question of what follows death; that is, the death of the corporeal body. Is there life after death? Is there a God or some other power, force, or intelligence to whom we must account for the conduct of our lives? Do we go to some heavenly realm, or to a hellish punishment? Are we born again, locked in an unending wheel of existence? Such questions are typical religious speculations. In the West their answers serve as the cornerstones of belief, and the answers that religions provide are the pillars of faith.

The Chinese are different. The pragmatic quality of traditional beliefs and attitudes is clearly seen in the Chinese attitude towards death. As is often the case, we must consider what is absent to understand and appreciate what is present. The Chinese pay no particular attention to an afterlife in the Western sense. This point is clearly made in the following passage from Lin Yu Tang's *My Country, My People.*

> *Nothing is more striking than the Chinese humanist devotion to the true end of life as they conceive it, and the complete ignoring of all theological or metaphysical phantasies extraneous to it. When our great humanist Confucius was asked about the important question of death, his famous reply was, "Don't know life—how know death?"*

To the Chinese, death is at once utterly simple and profoundly mysterious; for death is simply the loss of *qì*, the separation of yīn and yáng.

In responding to the passing of loved ones, the Chinese tend not to explain or rationalize the loss. They simply grieve for it. But they attend to the continuation of the social relationships, the underlying bonds on which family and society depend. The respect of time-honored customs in the worship of the departed is seen in the long and attenuated funeral observances. Thus even in death, the power of *qì* to permeate and connect all the facets of Chinese life can be observed. As those who have died surrender their *qì* to the "Great *Qì*" of nature, those who survive absorb the absence of the dead and fill the void with their own emotion and devotion to the Chinese way of life.

By focusing on death, we can see that the Chinese have evolved a pattern of belief and behavior that reveals important cultural values. The values they place on life are clearly reflected in their behavior concerning the dead. In mourning the death of loved ones, the Chinese openly and frankly express their grief. Conversely, and in some ways paradoxically, they also observe elaborate yet subtle rituals as they grieve, both publicly and privately.

How can we understand Chinese beliefs, attitudes and behaviors concerning death as a background to the theories and practices of traditional Chinese medicine? First and foremost we must recognize that the traditional definition of death is the loss of *qì*. Doctors of Chinese medicine pay particular attention to the patient's *qì*, but in patients who are near death, this becomes a matter of the utmost vigilance. The worst possible sign is a sudden, apparent resurgence of *qì*, because this is often observed in critically ill patients just before they die. In Chinese medicine this is known as "the candle burning brightly before it is extinguished."

The idea of *qì* in the relationship between life and death is particularly illuminated by comparison to attitudes in the West. The following is taken from *Death in Han China* by Kenneth Brashier regarding Han (221–207 B.C.E.) attitudes about death.

> *One common example of this evocation process is the deceased's age at death. In the elegiac hymn, a child may be the "bud that never blossomed," a young man may "fall down in his morning" and an old woman may simply "return forever to her darkened hovel." For the actual age at death, the rememberer must recall the preface details where it is almost always recorded. At first glance, remembering this detail may seem of negligible importance in preserving*

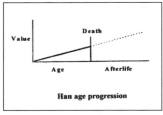

Figure 2

identity, but the ancestor's final age is vital in Han culture that regards children as not yet human and mandates veneration of the elderly. *Affecting everything from the seating order at village feasts to the mitigation of punishments, age is a key factor in determining how an ancestor ties into the rest of the social order [Fig 2]. Advanced age is even regarded as a sign of moral integrity.*

This contrasts with Western experience. According to George Minois' "History of Old Age: From Antiquity to the Renaissance," Westerners envision the steps of life as an arc, peaking at forty or fifty and declining toward a "devalued old age," a visualization that is found in both literature and art since at least Dante's time. A recent study entitled "Celebrations of Death: The Anthropology of Mortuary Ritual" reveals that little has changed: "The life of the individual

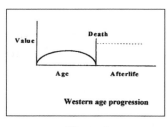

Figure 3

should rise in an arc through brassy youth to fruitful middle years, and then decline gently toward a death that is acceptable as well as inevitable." At the point of death, Christianity would extend this arc, causing it to "resurge"—the Latin derivation of "resurrection." Thus, Western age progression has the shape of Figure 3.

In contrast, the Han Chinese envisioned age progression in a significantly different manner. As already noted, at one end children were relatively unvalued and at the other, the elderly enjoyed the highest status. As for death, both surviving Han literature and modern archaeology stress continuity, even to the point of asking the dead how they spend each night and designing their tombs to resemble abodes for living. That afterdeath existence is likened to a series of promotions into larger and larger groups; as the dead increase in rank, they paradoxically lose their identity within the ancestral crowd. As they fade from memory, sacrifices to them become increasingly rare, but because they are rare, they are more esteemed.

The value of such etic graph-making rests in the questions that appear where the graphs differ. For example, the well-demarcated

WHO CAN RIDE THE DRAGON?

"point of death" on the Western graph is replaced by a less distinctive "process of death" on the Han graph, a fact the surviving Han stelae amply confirm. At the end of life in the Western age progression, the shift from devalued old age to afterlife requires a fantastic leap, a radical transformation. At the end of life in the Han age progression, there is only a subtle transformation as the world begins to darken and as the recent ancestors' qì merges with the original qì from which their life, and all others, condensed. From that point onward the dead undergo the structured amnesia of gradually fading away.

Finally, in both graphs the period directly before death affects the period after death. Where the Western graph requires the mysterious transformation to reclaim lost ground, the Han graph carries on its ascent. In other words, the value placed on aging directly bears upon afterlife beliefs. Understanding Han ancestral remembrance explains the Han attitude toward aging.

The Chinese medical understanding of death is deceptively simple. When yīn and yáng can no longer sustain their complex interrelationship, when the qì no longer surges and circulates between the yīn and yáng of the body, the body ceases to live. Yet this simple explanation underlies a complex array of attitudes and beliefs about life and death in traditional Chinese religion and philosophy. We will examine some of these ideas in the next chapter, for they have influenced all aspects of life in ancient China.

For now, it is sufficient to say that the "children of the dragon" developed a simple and pragmatic attitude: to take whatever steps were possible to lengthen life and maintain youth. According to the theories of Chinese medicine, this can only be accomplished by conserving and cultivating the harmony of yīn and yáng so that the qì that arises from them can flow, continuously preserving life's treasures. As we have seen, this potent metaphor of incessant transformation permeates Chinese beliefs, myths, and customs. Ever since it escaped from Pán Gǔ's giant egg, the qì of heaven and earth has served as the root of Chinese life. It is the priceless treasure of Chinese culture. It also serves as the basis for much of Chinese philosophy and religion.

CHAPTER THREE

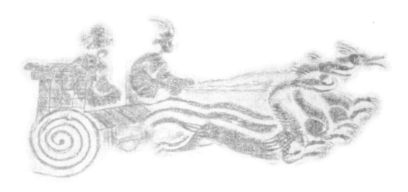

 Philosophy and Religion

To the West, it seems hardly imaginable that the relationship between man and man (which is morality) could be maintained without reference to a Supreme Being, while to the Chinese it is equally amazing that men should not, or could not, behave toward one another as decent beings without thinking of their indirect relationship through a third party.

—LIN YU TANG

It is difficult to imagine two human activities that are seemingly more opposite in nature than medicine and religion. Religion requires blind faith and unswerving devotion to ideology. To be suitable for faith, religious theories must be unprovable. Medicine, on the other hand, demands theories that reliably yield pragmatic and demonstrable results. In fact, in medicine, "proof" is defined as statistical probability. Where people may demonstrate faith by dying for their religious beliefs, the devotion of medical people is to saving lives, and doctors cannot limit themselves to ideas that conform to a particular creed. They must be free to follow the theories and methods they know to work. Yet as we read the history of Chinese medicine we can observe how closely religion and philosophy were entwined with medicine.

Like their counterparts in other cultures, Chinese philosophers and priests, whether Buddhist, Daoist, or Confucian, evolved elaborate explanations of life's meaning and mysteries. Chinese doctors carefully studied any wisdom that might help them to better understand the nature of life and how to rescue it from disease. In part because of the distinctively philosophical nature of Chinese religion, Chinese doctors discovered important theoretical principles in religious writing and incorporated these into the foundations of traditional Chinese medical theory.

Thus we uncover a rich and complex layer in the cultural substrate of Chinese medicine: philosophy and religion. Although we cannot hope to exhaust the material available, we can sample and savor the essence of China's three major religions as we seek to understand how these ideas and beliefs influenced and supported the development of medicine.

There is an indigenous tradition of "religion" in China that dates to earliest antiquity. To some extent, traditional Chinese ways of religious observance are expressed in how the Chinese people conduct their lives, regardless of the ideology or dogma they chose to follow. As observed by Lin Yu Tang in the quote that begins this chapter, this Chinese approach to religion is distinctly different from custom in the Western world. This applies to Buddhists, Daoists, and even Chinese Christians, Jews, and Moslems. There are, of course, doctrinal variations between religious faiths and schools of thought in China. Some of these are subtle, some obvious; some are minor, some fundamental. Yet such variations serve to underscore the invariably Chinese undercurrent of belief that infuses Chinese religious ideology and methodology.

The same can be said of philosophy. Indeed, much of China's religious tradition is rooted in philosophical sources. For example, it is not entirely possible to differentiate Daoist religion from Daoist philosophy in Chinese history. Today, it is somewhat easier, although lines of demarcation between the religion and the philosophy are easily washed away by the flow of ideas and practices. Moreover, an eclectic spirit has flourished throughout China's long history and intellectuals have mingled the tenets of philosophies and faiths into what has been called the "religion of common sense."

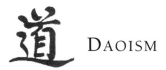 DAOISM

Of all the religious and philosophical traditions of China, none is more typically Chinese than the school of thought known as Daoism. With roots in the most ancient traditions and beliefs, it first emerged as a cohesive set of precepts and principles in the period of the Warring States (475–221 B.C.E.). Its central theme is the *dào*. *Dào* is virtually impossible to translate with a single English word. It means many things: "path, road, avenue, method, way." But none of its denotations begin to explain its deepest philosophical meanings. Neither are the difficulties of understanding the meaning of Daoism limited to the problem of translation. The "bible" of Daoism begins with an obtuse warning to those who seek to follow this way: "The *Dào* that can be spoken is not the eternal *Dào*."

The character itself, 道, is somewhat enigmatic. It is composed of two elements. The first is the character for "head," *shǒu* 首. The second is *zhǒu*, a character that means "walk" or "go," which appears as ⻌ when it is used as an element in a compound character. Combining these two meanings presents an idea of "the head in motion," which, in fact, approximates one of the definitions of *dào*, "to think."

Its meaning as a philosophical term can be understood as knowing the way to go, of engaging the head in motion. In the philosophy of Daoism this notion of using one's head to move was extraordinarily developed. As a philosophical concept, understanding the *dào* came to mean wisdom about the entire way of existence, its origin, its principles, its direction or aim, and even its ineffable mysteries.

Like many traditions in China, the origins of Daoism are traced to a figure obscured by legend and antiquity. Lao Zi, the Librarian of the State of Lu, spent his youth trying to persuade his peers and state officials of the practical value of his naturalistic philosophy. "Ruling a country," wrote the sage, "is like cooking a small fish." If you've cooked enough small fish, the meaning is clear. The more you do—the more elaborate your cooking methods—the more likely you are to ruin the meal. Lao Zi's logic proposed that "doing nothing" was far more efficacious than "striving to win the world." But few heeded what seemed an arcane and esoteric magic. Legend has it that Lao Zi, despairing of finding disciples, retired from civilization. Along the way he stopped to record his thoughts in a 5000-word treatise known as the *Dào Dé Jīng* or *Classic of the Dào and Dé*. The word *dé* is somewhat less problematic than *dào*. It means "moral" or "moral virtue."

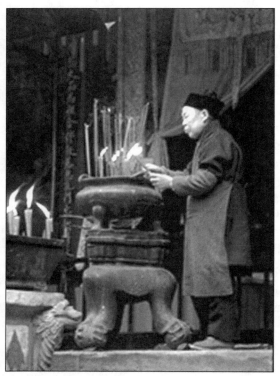

A Daoist nun at Tian Shi Dong (Temple of the Heavenly Teacher) on Qing Cheng Mountain tends the burnt offerings in the temple courtyard

In fact, Lao Zi's teachings, as recorded in the *Dào Dé Jīng* and transmitted from generation to generation with all the pomp and ceremony of any orthodoxy, are rooted in a single term that baffles and bemuses his followers to this day: *wú wéi*, "non-action." Only through non-action, reasoned the venerable sage, could one harmonize with the constant change of nature. He chose water as his primal image, for in its constant seeking of low and lower places in its cyclic journey to the sea, water exhibits what Lao Zi treasured as the most priceless principle of conduct: no resistance.

Why is the sea the King of all streams? Because it lies lower than they.

In the softness and yielding nature of water, Lao Zi divined the hidden and mysterious power of nature. His whole philosophy can be understood as a guide to those who seek to comprehend and harmonize with this mystery. In Chapter 25 of the *Dào Dé Jīng* we read:

> *There are four phenomena of greatness in the universe; mankind is one of them. Mankind follows the ways of the earth. The earth follows the ways of heaven. Heaven follows the ways of the Dào. Dào follows the ways of Nature.*

"*Dào* follows the ways of Nature." We find this inscription carved and painted in gold letters of the finest script above the doorways of Daoist shrines and temples throughout China. This yearning for harmony with the natural world and with the phenomena of nature was the organizing principle around which both the Daoist philosophy and religion developed, and develop they did. In the ensuing centuries, Daoism became an elaborate amalgamation of sorcery, spirit worship, alchemy, and esoterica. For this Way of Nature led Daoists to the "gateway of all indescribable marvels" enshrouded by "mystery upon mystery."

The first organized Daoist group was established in the Eastern Han period by an individual known as Zhang Dao Lin in the year 142 C.E. He chose a mountain in what is now Sichuan Province as his home. He Min Shan, Crane's Call Mountain, became the center of China's first formal Daoist cult. Hundreds and thousands of followers flocked to the mountain, each paying a tribute of five bushels of rice. The sect became known as the "Five Bushels of Rice Cult."

Zhang Dao Lin was not only a philosopher, he was an exponent of a school of thought that stressed the importance of sexual cultivation in order to treat disease, attain longevity, and perform the ultimate magical act and accomplish the aim of alchemy: immortality. We know from materials unearthed at the Ma Wang Dui tombs that such concepts were well-formulated by the second millennium B.C.E. By that time they had also become infused in the earliest extant texts on medical theory, such as the *Yellow Emperor's Canon of Internal Medicine*.

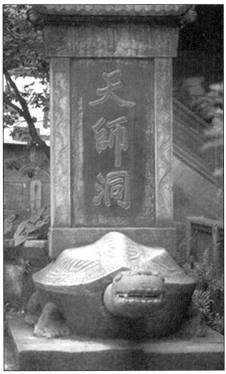

A tortoise carved in stone carries the nameboard of the Temple of the Heavenly Teacher (Tian Shi Dong) on Qing Cheng Mountain

Though the specific activities of these early Daoists are difficult to deduce from historical records, it seems clear that they practiced a number of methods classified under the heading of *yăng shēng*. The basic meaning of this term is "cultivate health." Many different practices were included: meditation, *qì gōng,* dietary disciplines including fasting, the use of various (mainly supplementing) herbs; and exercises known as *dǎo yǐn.* Foremost among these practices was a series of sexual techniques designed to cultivate and preserve the *jīng,* or "essence."

The Five Bushels of Rice cult eventually died out, but its practices survived. By the Sui and Tang dynasties (581 C.E.–907 C.E.), such health practices had developed into a tradition of Daoist alchemy known as the "Golden Elixir." Daoist alchemists were seminal figures in classifying the herbal, mineral, and animal ingredients used in Chinese medical formulas. Their experimentation to develop an elixir of eternal life produced an enormous body of empirical knowledge of how to apply numerous medicinal substances.

Throughout its more than 2500-year history, the subject of Daoism has provided medical students with far more than a lifetime's study. Lao Zi's esoteric, magical view of man's ideal relationship with nature influenced the early medical theorists whose work endures as the cornerstone of medical practice.

In his *Prescriptions Worth A Thousand Pieces of Gold,* the great Tang Dynasty alchemist and physician Sun Si Miao wrote: "If you do not study Lao Zi and Zhuang Zi, you will not know how to live your life from day to day." To understand the implications of such a remark, we need to concentrate on the associations found among the constellation of ideas that form the theoretical infrastructure of Chinese medicine.

In the *Yellow Emperor's Canon of Internal Medicine,* there is an important point made near the end of the "Treatise on the Interaction of Yīn and Yáng." This treatise covers important aspects of mankind's relationship with the natural world, especially harmonization with the movements in the world that correspond to the changes of the seasons (i.e. the transformation of *qì*). This famous passage provides the definition of the superior doctor: one who treats his patients before they get ill. One implication of this text is clearly derived from Daoist roots: the ability to prevent disease can only come from living one's life in harmony with the forces of nature.

The Chinese of antiquity understood the vital necessity of being in harmony with the time of year, the time of day, and as well with the various periods of one's life. This sensibility to changes in time, weather, and other natural phenomena went far beyond a simple sense of knowing when to plant and when to harvest. Early geomancers associated the affairs of people with the movement of the stars, the planets, the seasons, the sun, the moon, the earth, and the creatures and forces living upon it.

To a large extent, the development of this whole sensibility into an articulate logic derives from the philosophy of Daoism. Daoist thinking stands as a unique structure in the cultural treasurehouse of ancient China. It is a crystallization of the antique wisdom that guided Lao Zi's ancestors through thousands of years of cultural growth and development. This is an extremely important point to comprehend in proper perspective. The philosophy of Daoism, although it originates some 2400 years ago, is a reflection of traditional thoughts about life that were already ancient when the legendary Lao Zi committed his words to ink.

Sun Si Miao was a prominent Daoist of his day. The great British sinologist, Joseph Needham, identifies him as the likely inventor of the formula for gunpowder. If it was Sun who discovered gunpowder, he likely came across it while experimenting to discover the elixir of eternal life, which was the preeminent concern of Daoist alchemists.

Writing a thousand years after Lao Zi, Sun Si Miao noted that through studying the writings of the Daoist philosophers, medical students would have a guide for harmonizing themselves with the world in which they live.

"Physician, heal thyself," goes the ancient Hippocratic saying. The Chinese version might read, "Physician, keep thyself in harmony with yīn and yáng thus denying death and disease untimely opportunities." This approach to preventive medicine lies at the heart of Chinese medicine. That such an attitude exists is directly attributable to the philosophical religion known as Daoism.

As if the contribution of this fundamental concern for natural harmony were not sufficient, the Daoists also provided Chinese medical theorists with important aspects of the concept of *qì*. To be sure, the concept of *qì* is far more ancient than the Daoist school of thought, but in Daoism, the notion of *qì* as the source of life and of life's continuation was developed and refined in a unique and comprehensive way.

In Chapter Ten of the *Dào Dé Jīng*, for example, Lao Zi poses an obscure yet intriguing series of questions:

> *Can one unify the spirit of the blood and the spirit of the breath and keep them from separating? In concentrating the qì to attain resiliency, can one be like a baby?*

The relationship between qì and blood lies at the very center of the ancient Chinese model of human physiology. The *Yellow Emperor's Canon* states, "The *qì* is the commander of the blood. The blood is the mother of the *qì*." It was Lao Zi and his followers who focused their attention on the mysterious and illusory nature of *qì* in search for insights into how life began and how it could be fostered and protected. Their insights proved invaluable to the development of medical theories and techniques.

The entire structure of the theory of yīn and yáng owes much of its form and contents to Daoism. The *Dào Dé Jīng* states, "All things bear yīn but embrace yáng, thus their pulsing qì unites." Nowhere in Chinese literature is the essence of the relationship between yīn, yáng, and *qì* more clearly defined than in such passages. Thus we see that the treasure-house of Chinese medicine stands on a foundation that was built by Daoist philosophers.

佛 CHINESE BUDDHISM

There have been few influences upon Chinese culture and intellectual development over the centuries that have been as significant or profound as that of Buddhism. However, its imprint on the theories of Chinese medicine is more subtle than that of Daoism or Confucianism.

The first Buddhist monks probably came from India to China in the 1st century C.E. This marked the opening of an era of intense exchange of people, customs, knowledge, and literature. For the next four or five centuries, large numbers of Buddhist sutras were translated into Chinese. The results of this high level of importation of Buddhist texts and ideas were complex and far-reaching.

In one important respect, the Buddhist religion established itself as an alternative to the native, naturalistic belief system which until then had perpetuated more or less without structure or organization. That is to say, prior to the arrival of Buddhism in China, there were no organized institutions of Daoism, for example, or of anything else. This is not to say that there were not significant bodies of philosophical and religious material. They had simply never served as the foundation for religious cults until the arrival of the Buddhists.

WHO CAN RIDE THE DRAGON?

Buddhist monks proselytized and attracted followers from among the Chinese populace, and as the size and number of such congregations increased, the indigenous philosophers and ideologues must have experienced pangs of competition. They turned to the forms and practices of this new religion for models, and soon the first Daoist cults appeared, for example, the Five Bushels of Rice Cult, noted earlier.

To an outsider viewing the temples of each religion for the first time, the resemblance between contemporary Daoist and Buddhist forms of worship seems obvious. However, there are distinguishing particulars of dress and hairstyle. Buddhist monks commonly shave their heads, whereas Daoists never cut their hair—both men and women wear it in a topknot, often beneath a characteristic close-fitting cap. Buddhists wear robes of saffron, purple, brown, and other colors; Daoists have chosen a monochromatic blue. To a foreigner, monks and nuns of either discipline appear otherwise rather similar, reflecting what we have termed the indigenous Chinese tradition of religious practice.

When Buddhism came into contact with Chinese culture and native religions, it underwent a long, slow, and profound evolution. The influences of Indian Buddhism and the indigenous philosophic religions of China moved in both directions. Not only did Daoism and to a lesser degree Confucianism take their organizational cues from the Buddhists, but Buddhism in China changed in important ways. Several themes have emerged in the ensuing centuries that characterize Chinese Buddhism and distinguish it from how it is observed and practiced in other countries.

First and foremost among these is the Chinese portrayal of Buddhist images and identities. In China, from the most ancient times onward, ancestors were deified. Thus, words like "god," or "spirit" are commonly interchangeable. There are many "gods" that populate a loose affiliation of spirits that includes people who have died and risen to the position of a god through the veneration bestowed upon them by their faithful heirs or followers. Such gods mingle freely with others who are more closely recognizable as Western notions of deity.

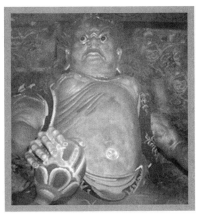

Statue of a fierce Boddhisatva at the Divine Light Monastery

The Buddhist hierarchy descends from the great Siddhartha Gautama and includes notable monks and lamas who through their meditation, compassion for others, teaching, and the examples of their lives have been rewarded with the title "Buddha." A display found in some of the larger Chinese Buddhist temples consists of 500 or more such Buddhas. There is a famous collection in the Divine Light Monastery just outside Chengdu.

Among the most venerated of these Buddhas in China is Guan Yin. The gender of this much loved and worshipped figure is ambivalent. Supposedly, the human being that was originally Guan Yin was a man. Yet this Buddha is almost always pictured as female. This may be from cultural associations with the primary attributes embodied by Guan Yin—mercy and compassion—which are bestowed upon the faithful.

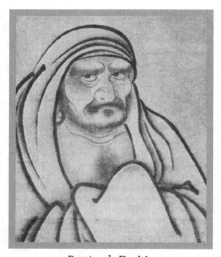
Patriarch Da Mo

One of the most significant contributions to Buddhism in China was begun by Bodhidharma, an Indian monk who came to China in the 4th century C.E. In China he came to be known as Da Mo Da Shi (the great teacher Da Mo). He lived an ascetic lifestyle and stressed a path to enlightenment characterized by strenuous, solitary meditation. According to legend, he spent nine years meditating in a mountain cave before he experienced awakening. He is widely respected throughout the Buddhist world and celebrated as the first patriarch of Zen Buddhism.

The school of Buddhism founded in China by Da Mo is known as Chan. This is a Chinese transliteration of the Hindu word *dhyana*. In Japanese it is pronounced "Zen." This form of Buddhism is characterized by sudden, complete, spiritual awakening resulting from strenuous adherence to the "method" or "way." This is the literal translation of *dhyana*. This "method" focuses on one main theme: it is all in your mind. Reality is illusion. The ultimate reality is Emptiness. This typically Buddhist idea was exquisitely refined in the teachings of Da Mo and his followers. It was an idea that ran contrary to the Chinese naturalistic and humanistic tendencies so vividly expressed in the teachings of the

WHO CAN RIDE THE DRAGON?

Daoists and the Confucians. By the 10th century this conflict had become institutionalized. Joseph Needham clearly pointed this out citing Hu Yin, a 10th century writer:

> Hu Yin, for example (+1093 to +1151), considered that ice and glowing coals would mix better than Confucianism and Buddhism. In the Sun Yuan Hsueh An, he is reported as saying, "Buddhism looks upon emptiness as the highest (khung wei chih) and upon existence as an illusion (yu we huan). Those who wish to learn the true Dào take good note of this. Daily we see the sun and moon revolving in the heavens, and the mountains and rivers rooted in the earth, while men and animals wander abroad in the world. If ten thousand Buddhas were to appear all at once, they would not be able to destroy the world, to arrest its movements, or to bring it to nothingness. The sun has made day and the moon night, the mountains have stood firm and the rivers have flowed, men and animals have been born since the beginning of time—these things have never changed, and one should rejoice that this is so. If one thing decays, another arises. My body will die, but mankind will go on. So all is not emptiness."

The opposition between Buddhism and the other schools of thought in China has provided the basis for numerous political, economic, as well as ideological conflicts through the centuries. From such conflicts there have emerged different approaches to many traditional Chinese studies and practices. For example, there are uniquely Buddhist traditions of qì gōng, herbal medicine, and health preservation that have developed over the centuries. Among the major contributions of Buddhism to Chinese medicine was the introduction of a number of Indian medicinal herbs and their uses. In fact, this movement of people and ideas brought a large number of herbal ingredients to China, both from India and other parts of the world. These include hóng huā (red flower), xuè jié (dragon's blood) and mǎ qián zǐ (nux vomica). Not only were such ingredients adopted but also the systematic correspondences used to categorize them in Indian texts were to some extent included in the overall Chinese scheme for categorizing materia medica.

A contemporary writer, Zhang Xiu Feng, points out:

> Buddhism did not originally strive for the preservation of life per se. But in fact, the practice of Buddhist meditation results in similar benefits. ... The final purpose of the study of Buddhism is to awaken

the heart and understand the true nature, to rid oneself of "what I hold on to" . . . to be set free from all manner of man-made disturbances and suffering.

At Wen Shu Yuan, Chengdu's largest Buddhist temple, the resident physician explained it to us as follows:

There is little direct relationship between Buddhism and medicine, not nearly as much as there is between Daoism and medicine. The purpose of Buddhism is to free people's souls. If the mind and soul are free, people don't suffer from disease, or from anything else.

Perhaps the most significant contribution of Buddhism to the intellectual establishment in China was the concept of "awakening," described above. The characteristic of Chinese Buddhist awakening or enlightenment is contained in the story of the sixth patriarch of Chan (Zen) Buddhism, Hui Neng. The story centers on the transmission of the *yī bō*. The first patriarch, Da Mo, gave his mantle (*yī*) and alms bowl (*bō*) to his chosen successor, the second patriarch, Hui Ke, as a symbol of succession to the leadership of the Chan sect. This legacy was preserved by third, fourth, and fifth patriarchs as each selected his successor. It was received by Hui Neng, the sixth patriarch, but after him, it was never passed down again.

The reason is that Hui Neng destroyed it, and the meaning of that destruction reflects the subtle refinement of the Chinese Buddhist notion of awakening. Hui Neng was an orphan. As a child he came to the Dong Chan (Eastern Zen) temple and became a disciple of the fifth patriarch, Hong Ren. Throughout Hui Neng's stay at the temple, he had the most humble position. His work consisted of sweeping the yard, chopping wood, husking rice, and so forth. One day, Hong Ren gathered all of his disciples and asked them each to compose a poem. Though he didn't reveal it at the time, Hong Ren was looking for his successor. His leading pupil, Shen Xiu, composed the following poem:

The body is the tree of bodhi (awakening). The heart is the plateau of the clear mirror. Whisk it diligently every moment, so that no dust can settle.

When the master read his pupil's poem, he realized that Shen Xiu had yet to cross the threshold and had only just arrived at the gateway of awakening. Finding no better composition, however, Hong Ren told the assembly that they could study Shen's poem and if they followed it, they could avoid the path of evil.

WHO CAN RIDE THE DRAGON?

Hui Neng could not study the poem, because he could not read. Thus, while the others were reading and musing over the poem, Hui Neng asked one of them to help him write his own thoughts down. He could not write them himself, for neither had he ever learned to write. The poem Hui Neng dictated read:

Originally, Bodhi had no tree.
The clear mirror has no plateau.
Originally, there is nothing.
Where can dust settle?

When the monks saw Hui Neng's poem, they were astonished. They brought it to Hong Ren saying that Hui Neng was on the road to awakening. Hong Ren read the poem and had nothing good to say about it. His only comment was that Hui Neng was not yet awakened. That evening, however, the patriarch called upon the disciple, taught him the Diamond Sutra, and gave him his *yī bō*. He explained that when Da Mo first came to China no one knew him and he had passed on this legacy so it could be handed down from generation to generation, as a symbol of authenticity. He pointed out that the true teaching could only be conducted from heart to heart, privately and secretly. He also warned Hui Neng that the *yī bō* had become an object of jealousy and controversy. He advised that it no longer be handed down. "If you pass it on, your life will be like a silk thread. You must leave this place at once. I'm afraid someone will harm you."

That night, the two of them left the temple in secrecy. As Hong Ren foresaw, the other disciples were furious when they learned that the mantle of their sect had been handed down to Hui Neng. They set out after him to recover it. Finally they caught up with him and demanded the mantle and the alms bowl, Hui Neng flung them to the ground. The earthen bowl shattered.

Hui Neng's teaching had a profound influence on the development of Chan Buddhism. He stressed that all that mattered was the practice of seated, silent meditation and the attainment of awakening. The true nature of life could not be contained in bowl or a mantle, nor could it be passed on from master to student, except in the way that he himself had received the teaching from his teacher, heart to heart.

Even the Neo-Confucians, such as Hu Yin, quoted above, though arguing against the ideology of the Buddhists, were greatly impressed with this concept of awakening and incorporated the notion of gaining enlightenment concerning the essence of a wide range of ideas in their approach to scholarship. Thus their interpretations of both Daoist and Confucian ideology included the idea that the truths of these philosophies could be "awakened" in those who diligently applied themselves to their study.

Although it is not possible to point out a direct relationship between Buddhist concepts and the theories of Chinese medicine, the flavor of Buddhist thinking has influenced the development and practice of medicine in China since the first Buddhist monks arrived. This influence is most notable in the practice of medical *qì gōng*. Many of the practitioners of medical *qì gōng* are Buddhists, and their cultivation of *qì* as an instrument of healing reflects the Buddhist concentration on purifying the senses and awakening the mind and spirit.

If the traces of Buddhism on Chinese medicine are faint and hard to follow, those of Confucianism, as we shall see next, stand out in high relief.

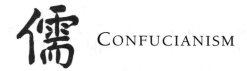 CONFUCIANISM

There is so much misunderstood, misperceived, mistakenly devalued, or discarded by Western observers of Chinese culture that it is impossible to say that one aspect or artifact is most misunderstood. However, were we to list the traditional Chinese subjects mistaken or misapprehended by non-Chinese, the subject of Confucius and the school of thought that bears his name would be near the top.

Most people in the Western world do not understand Confucianism beyond the fortune cookie aphorisms frequently acquired at the end of a trip to the Chinese restaurant for *moo goo gai pan*. "A refreshing change is coming in the near future." "Waste not, want not." It is the "No tick-ee no washee" school of chauvinized Confucianism that many Westerners attend. Perhaps it's not quite that bad, but, then again, perhaps it is! To comprehend the nature of Chinese culture and society, much less its indigenous medicine, we must develop an articulate understanding of Confucian influence.

The social contract in China contains a fair number of clauses that reached their most eloquent expression in works of the Confucian school. And, as we shall see, these principles of social organization and administration found their way directly into medical theory and practice.

On its surface, Confucian doctrine appears as trite homilies concerned with harmonizing household and empire alike by focusing on "right action," the observance of antique rituals, and the strict observation of traditional social hierarchies. A closer look reveals a compelling and compassionate humanism, summed by a memorable quote attributed to the late *tài jí* master Zheng Man Qing, who referred to himself as a follower of "The Master": "I never wanted to be a buddha or god. I only wanted to be a man."

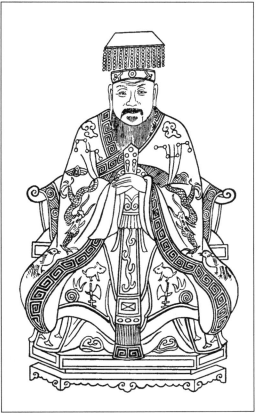

Woodcut of Confucius in court dress

Delving deeper into Confucian texts we discover a profound metaphysics and a coordinated system that rationalizes the human condition and provides broad models of self cultivation and social development. Among these Confucian ideals none is more important than the hierarchy of relationships interlacing all human affairs. This concept of a social hierarchy has had a profound influence on Chinese culture, or more specifically, on the Chinese state of mind.

One thing that becomes clear to anyone who spends time living with Chinese people is that they tend to enter into social relations with precepts of where and how they belong that are considerably different than those of Westerners. The American "state of mind," for example, includes an important element of "independent spirit." Americans quest, even today, for independence in their hearts and in their minds. "I did it my way." "Don't tread on me." "A man's home is his castle." All are trite and perhaps dated expressions of an American vision that time has worn thin in the closing days of the twentieth century. Yet all these statements make reference to this vital spirit of America: to be free and independent.

The millennia-old tradition of Chinese civilization runs, if not contrary to the American spiritual vector, at least at a divergent angle. For the traditional Chinese, the synthesis of an accurate and functional concept of where they fit in the social hierarchy is a far more pressing question than freedom and independence. The various relative positions are all well known, and are easily observable by both outward and inward signs. These positions tend to subsume those who occupy them.

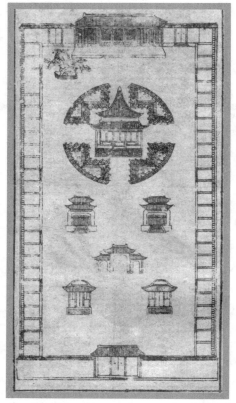

The Confucian layout of a typical courtyard

This does not imply a lack of individuality in the Chinese spirit; indeed, the Chinese are fiercely individualistic. Yet their common understanding of the value and importance of social positions and relationships contributes to a characteristic pattern of expression. In traditional society the extent to which anyone fully expresses his or her individuality is clearly understood as a reflection of their power.

Only the Emperor could wear yellow of the imperial hue. The Emperor's gate faced to the south, the most propitious of the four cardinal points. The Emperor's throne was the farthest seat from the door, and always facing it—the position of highest honor. Even the design of their clothing, the height and cut of their collars, and the shape of their headgear, revealed the Chinese individual's place in this hierarchy.

The list of particulars goes on and on. It is a list which is reflected in daily life in China to the present day. It is the elaborate and well understood code of social conduct. For example, the guest of honor at a banquet is always seated furthest from the door. A host cannot but offer tea and snacks to a visitor, and the visitor is similarly bound to refuse such offers. The host must persist and the guest must persevere until after observing

WHO CAN RIDE THE DRAGON?

three such rounds of Confucian etiquette, he or she can at last surrender and accept hospitality.

The Emperor, son of heaven, stands at the very peak of this social hierarchy. We say "stands" rather than "stood" because regardless of the political ideology in vogue in China's capital, the position of China's leaders endures today as it has throughout Chinese civilization. Since set in place by China's first Emperor, it is not the mandate of Man's law that bestows ultimate power on the Emperor. It is the mandate of Heaven, of all the force and power that exists, that empowers the leader of China. It is a force that must be firmly grasped and wisely administered. It is a power that is widely coveted and cleverly sought by those few who deem themselves worthy of wielding it. It far exceeds the merely legalistic political power of a president or statesman.

This power depends on the heavenly principle *lǐ* as set forth in the works of Zhu Xi, a philosopher of the Song Dynasty who collected and revised the Confucian classics and formulated the school of thought that came to be known as Neo-Confucianism. At the core of this recapitulation of Chinese knowledge stood the "heavenly principle" or *lǐ*, which for the first time in Chinese intellectual history supplanted *qì* as the most basic principle of existence. It was this implicate order that gave rise to all existence according to the neo-Confucians.

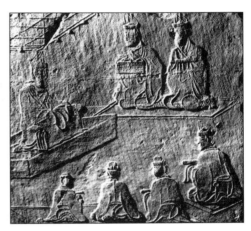

A Han Dynasty stone carving depicting Confucian scholars engaged in colloquy

Lǐ became the fundamental principle of Chinese philosophy. By the end of the thirteenth century, the work of Zhu Xi had gained such prominence that it served as the standard of instruction and examination in China's civil service system. The Emperor's power derived directly from this heavenly principle, and with this principle and power in place, he could subjugate all others and thus rule effectively.

The Emperor of China was not only the Son of Heaven. He was as well the father of the Empire and of all its subjects. He ministered to his progeny and saw to their wellbeing through an extensive and elaborate hierarchy of assistants. These all existed to forward their leader's power and thereby shared it to some extent. They never approached the omnipotence of the emperor himself. His was an absolute state, attended by absolute rules.

This social contract was fashioned, in large part, by the scions of the Confucian school. Chinese citizens throughout the centuries have accepted it for the great benefits that it bestows upon them. These benefits can be summed in a single word: order—or, at least, the semblance of order. The Chinese are a boisterous and exuberant people. Only a few days in China will disabuse most first-time travelers of the notion of the diffident Oriental. The Chinese work hard and play hard. But they toil within a well-conceived and well-established social framework that provides them a constant sense of where they belong in the scheme of things. It is a scheme derived in large part from the philosophy of Confucius.

It is no surprise to find at the heart of the science of Chinese medical formula composition a principle that is entirely derived from the Confucian model of society. To function effectively, an herbal prescription needs to contain not only the right ingredients, in the right proportions, it must be elegantly balanced from several points of view. Foremost among these are the relative roles that each ingredient plays. This is described by a metaphor that compares each constituent to an analogous position in the courtly hierarchy.

A formula is seen to have a "sovereign" herb, one that commands the overall direction and function of the medicine. There are "ministerial" constituents, those that assist the sovereign in accomplishing the medicianl aim, as well as couriers or guides that lead the other ingredients to their intended targets within the body's systems. This theoretical principle is contained in the phrase, "jūn chén zuǒ shǐ."

These words are taken directly from terms that designate positions of descending rank in the imperial court. Jūn is the highest rank, the soverign or commander. Chén is the minister, the close companion and advisor of the ruler. Zuǒ is the assistant, an attache or adjuvant. Shǐ is the courier. In an herbal formula these are often ingredients that direct the action of the prescription to a particular organ or system, just as a messenger delivers a message. This is not of course a summary of formula writing. It merely illustrates how deeply the concepts of Confucian social order penetrate, if only metaphorically, into the theoretical infrastructure of traditional medicine.

The first use of the terms jūn chén zuǒ shǐ did not, in fact, relate to formula writing, but to individual medicinals. In the earliest book devoted to herbology, the *Medicinal Canon of Shen Nong,* written in the

WHO CAN RIDE THE DRAGON?

Eastern Han (25–220 C.E.), herbs were classified into several "grades" reflecting their comparative efficacy. Herbs of the highest grade were termed *jūn*, those of middle grade *chén*, while herbs of lower grade were known as *zuǒ* or *shǐ*.

This is just one example of how Confucian thinking influenced Chinese medicine. It is most important to recognize that Confucian thinking has permeated the thoughts of medical experts in China throughout history and is pervasive throughout Chinese medical theories.

The heart is termed the sovereign of the organs and the whole picture of human anatomy is presented in distinctly Confucian terms in almost every classical medical text. The concept of health itself is closely related to the well-ordered harmony that is the ideal of Confucian philosophy. A comprehensive plan of this anatomical harmony appears in Chapter Eight of the *Sù Wèn* portion of the Ilza Veith translation of the *Yellow Emperor's Canon of Internal Medicine:*

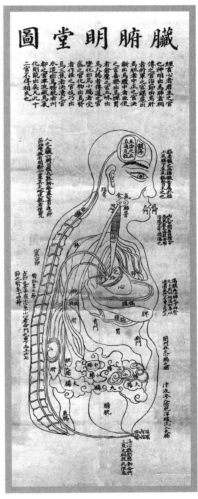

Chart of the internal organs described in the Yellow Emperor's Canon of Internal Medicine

> *The heart is like the minister or the monarch who excels through insight and understanding.*
>
> *The lungs are the symbol of the interpretation and conduct of the official jurisdiction and regulations.*
>
> *The liver has the functions of a military leader who excels in his strategic planning.*
>
> *The gallbladder occupies the position of an important and upright official who excels through his decisions and judgment.*
>
> *The middle of the thorax [the "center" or part between the breasts] is like the official of the center who guides the subjects in their joys and pleasures.*
>
> *The stomach acts as the official of the public granaries and grants the five tastes.*
>
> *The lower intestines are like the officials who propagate the Right Way of Living and generate evolution and change.*

The small intestines are like the officials who are trusted with riches, and they create changes of the physical substance.

The kidneys are like the officials who do energetic work, and they excel through their ability and cleverness.

The triple burner [a "virtual" organ system having a variety of functions but lacking an organic form] is like the officials who plan the construction of ditches and sluices, and create waterways.

The groins and the bladder are like the magistrates of a region or a district; they store the overflow and the fluid secretions which serve to regulate vaporization.

Here we see an orderly plan of the operation of the body in terms taken from the social and administrative structures of Chinese civilization. These structures, in turn, derive from the principles of Confucian logic. Though these principles were largely ignored by the rulers of Confucius' day, they provided subsequent generations of Chinese officials and scholars the accepted blueprint for social and medical order.

The "religion of common sense," as Lin Yu Tang called it, which developed in many schools of thought throughout Chinese history, has always been characterized by a spirit of eclecticism. Nowhere was this eclectic approach more prominent than in the relationship between the various philosophical and religious ideologies and medicine.

Indeed, one of the characteristics that distinguishes Chinese medicine from conventional Western medicine is its reliance on philosophical concepts as organizing principles to understand the body, health, and disease. Thus an understanding of the religious and philosophical roots of these principles is, as pointed out over a thousand years ago by the eminent Tang Dynasty physician, Sun Si Miao, a prerequisite for the study of medicine.

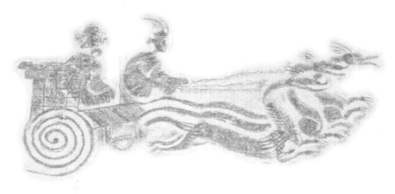

CHAPTER FOUR

文 *The Literary Tradition*

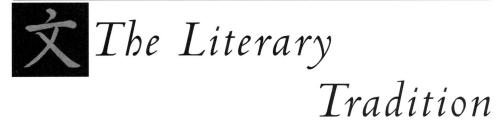

Our poems will be handed down with those of great dead poets. We can console ourselves. At least we shall have descendants.

—DU FU

My library was dukedom large enough.

—SHAKESPEARE

THE CHINESE ARE A LITERATE PEOPLE. This is not to say that there is no illiteracy in China, but to emphasize the elevated place afforded works of language and literature in traditional Chinese culture. Moreover, because of the aesthetics of Chinese words, Chinese literary and pictorial arts are intricately interwoven. Illustrated poems, paintings with poetic explanations, and particularly calligraphy—the pictorial realization of the essence of Chinese characters—are all to the present day highly treasured artistic forms.

Western nations also express high regard for literary works and those who create them. To achieve a sense of how the literary values of East and West compare, consider the following two stories. The first is a story about a great French writer, the second the legend of a Chinese poet.

A friend related the following story about lunch with Nobel laureate Albert Camus. "I'll tell you," began our friend, an Italian actor, "how the French are crazy for their writers."

I was to meet Camus at 12:30 at Maxim's in Paris. I arrived half an hour early. While I waited, I noticed a commotion at the entrance. The Maître d' and the head waiter were making a fuss over a customer who had just arrived. That customer turned out to be Phillipe Rothschild, then one of the wealthiest and most powerful men in Europe. With some commotion, the Baron was escorted to his regular table, and the staff resumed their routine duties.

A few minutes later, Camus appeared in the doorway. You've never seen anything like it. This time, the entire staff, including the chefs and the kitchen staff, dropped what they were doing and formed a receiving line, ten to fifteen people long, both sides of the door. They applauded as Camus made his way to the table where I was waiting. It was only then that I understood how crazy the French are for their writers.

Many in the West are familiar with the ceremonial dragon boat races that take place every spring in China or anywhere in the world where Chinese people live in significant numbers. Westerners recognize these dragon boats as characteristic symbols of Chinese culture and life. Yet, few realize that the festival surrounding the dragon boats celebrates the life and death of the great Warring States poet, Qu Yuan.

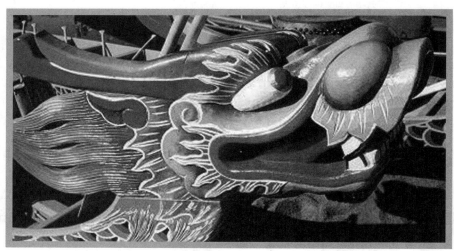

*The ornate and colorful carving of a modern-day dragon boat
(photo courtesy of Alvin Wang)*

Qu Yuan was not only a poet, but a statesman. Like so many of China's luminary minds, he was not appreciated in his own day. He served as the

Who Can Ride the Dragon?

Prime Minister of the state of Chu and sought, unsuccessfully, to engineer a political alliance with the neighboring state of Qi to resist the powerful Qin. It was the Qin king who later unified all of the warring states to form the Chinese empire.

Qu Yuan suffered from political intrigues and was twice banished during the course of his political career. When the Qin occupied the capital of Chu, Qu Yuan despaired of ever being able to return to his homeland and save it from the conquering Qin. On the fifth day of the fifth month in 278 B.C.E., Qu Yuan, clutching a heavy stone, threw himself into the Mi Luo River and drowned. For over 2000 years, every fifth of May according to the ancient lunar calendar, Chinese people everywhere throw rice dumplings called *zòng zǐ* into rivers to feed the fish so that they will not devour Qu Yuan's body. They stage the famous dragon boat races to scare evil spirits away from their drowned poet, who recorded his desperation in the epilogue of his famous poem, "Encountering Sorrow":

> *Forget it! No one in this country understands me. There is no reason, but I must cherish the homeland. There is no one to appreciate the ideal policy, so I am going to follow Peng Xian home.*

Peng Xian was a poet and statesman who lived several centuries earlier and threw himself into a river in despair of realizing lofty aims for his country. The deaths of both men exemplify a potent theme in Chinese literature and life: the ultimate sacrifice as a demonstration of undying devotion to the life of the homeland. The celebration of Qu Yuan's death is one of the most important festivals of the year, a festival for a poet who has been dead more than 2000 years. There is no comparable observance in the Western world, events such as a 1960's Parisian lunch notwithstanding.

Recently in Mexico there was a formal state funeral when Octavio Paz passed away. But will Mexicans memorialize Paz's death after 2000 years, or even ten? James Joyce, arguably one of the most influential writers of the twentieth century, was born on February 2. In the United States on February 2, people celebrate Groundhog Day. In the West, even the Bard himself is poorly remembered by comparison to Chinese veneration of Qu Yuan. When was Shakespeare's birthday? What day did he die and under what circumstances? Where few in the English speaking world could answer, or care, every schoolchild in China knows the story of Qu Yuan.

The virtual deification of the poet Qu Yuan is just one example of the unique status afforded to poets in traditional China, illustrating the extremely important role that Chinese literature plays in the lives of Chinese people. Not only have these traditions had a profound influence on Chinese art and culture generally, they have played a fundamental role in the development of traditional medical theory through 2000 years.

Despite the fact that no Chinese author has ever been awarded a Nobel Prize in literature, the literary tradition in China is home to some of the most exquisite, most lucid, and most compelling writing ever authored on Earth. There are explanations for the lack of recognition awarded Chinese writers by Westerners. Many, again, are problems of translation.

The problems of translating the literary art of the Chinese language are overwhelming. Image and meaning, sound and sense are intricately and delicately interwoven. Moreover, the pattern of the weave is all-important, just as the pattern of the strokes of a single character determine its shape, its sound, and its significance. As the Chinese put it when describing literary excellence, "There is a painting in the poem." Too often, once the interwoven sound, sense, shape, and feelings have been unraveled in translation, all that remains are meaningless threads. We are left wondering, "What do they mean?" We are reminded of the dilemma to which the great jazz musician Louis Armstrong referred in answer to the question, "What is jazz?" His answer: "If you gotta ask, you'll never know."

The study of China's literary tradition poses not simply a great difficulty; it offers an insight into the minds that conceived and composed the ancient works that inform Chinese medical theory. In fact, much of the basic theory of medicine in China is recorded in classical books that are works both of medical science and literature. Thus to understand and appreciate them we must devote some time and attention to the Chinese literary arts. Like all works of art, to be understood properly, a Chinese medical classic must be perceived and understood within the context of its origins.

Here we see another stark contrast between the study of Chinese medicine and conventional medical studies in the West. The scientific tradition of past centuries in the Western world has emphasized the segregation of scientific disciplines from both the liberal and fine arts. It is only recently that Westerners have begun to question the wisdom of imposing categorical separation between the disciplines of the arts and sciences.

The traditions of learning in China are quite opposite to those in Western universities. In traditional China, a comprehensive, integrative, and generalist approach to study has prevailed since ancient times. This is reflected in the traditional notion of a "master of many excellences." Such "excellences" frequently included poetry, calligraphy, painting, medicine, and martial arts. The Chinese ideal of a well-educated individual is far closer to the Western concept of a "renaissance man" than to the highly specialized experts who populate contemporary Western academia. Foremost among the skills that a man of learning had to master in traditional China were the correct and creative use of language. These included not simply basic literacy, but the use of the brush to calligraph characters, and an understanding of the literary and poetic forms used in the course of instruction and in civil service examinations.

Thus appreciation of the traditions from which they spring is a prerequisite for understanding these literary and medical classics. To do this, we must first understand what a book is in China and how books have functioned throughout Chinese history.

The oldest books in China were not originally books at all. Scratched on stone or bones, or burned into the shells of tortoises, the earliest recordings of literary composition in China are thousands of years old. These ancient glyphs and characters form the basis of many traditions of study and practice and are still lively subjects of study both in China and around the world. The oldest "texts" of China's earliest literary classic, the Yì Jīng, for example, were written on "oracle bones" in an ancient script known as jiá gū wén.

Many of the oldest extant copies of several texts we have mentioned, for example, the *Yellow Emperor's Canon of Internal Medicine,* the *Dào Dé Jīng,* and others, were scrolls made of bamboo and wooden slats, bound together with silk cords. Copies of many of these antique books were discovered in 1973 at a site known as Ma Wang Dui. Such books must have been scarce in 168 B.C.E. when the tombs at Ma Wang Dui were sealed, because China's first emperor had ordered the entire contents of all libraries burned some sixty years earlier. Medical books, the Yì Jīng, and a few other specific titles, escaped this imperial edict, one of the world's most ambitious attempts to revise history by burning it.

With the development of the technologies of paper-making in the Eastern Han (25–220 C.E.) and printing in the Song (960–1279 C.E.), books began to take on more recognizable forms. More importantly, the advent of these technologies allowed books to be copied, circulated, and therefore more readily studied.

Despite efforts like the book burnings of China's first emperor, the literary tradition survived and developed throughout China's imperial era. At the heart of this tradition is the notion of the Classic. What is a Classic? The word, in Chinese, is *jīng*. Curiously, this is the same *jīng* that figures so prominently in Chinese medical theory as the term for the channels (*jīng luò*) through which *qì* circulates throughout the body. *Jīng* means "to include, to manage or deal in; constant, regular; to pass through; warp [as in the warp of fabric]; longitude; as a result of." Applied to works of literature, *jīng* refers to those that have become constants or classics as a result of having succeeded from generation to generation. As they passed from era to era through Chinese history, these classics collected commentaries, revisions, and various other amendments.

A "Chinese classic" is thus an aggregation of material. We can seldom be sure of the authorship of such works. Writers of a later period often attributed their work to earlier authors, whose famous names would lend credibility to their work. Even written "evidence," therefore, of when, where, and from whom a particular work derives leaves many questions unanswered. The scholarship required to investigate such questions is considerable. Yet, generation after generation, the Classics continue their process of transmitting information that the Chinese continue to find indispensable.

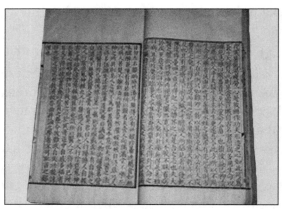

Text pages from a Chinese medical classic

WHO CAN RIDE THE DRAGON?

Indispensable, yes. Immutable, no. Successive generations tend to alter the contents of these literary classics, here adding, here taking away, according to a variety of criteria. Changing political climates give rise to scholarly reinterpretations. Development and refinement of technologies permitted closer scrutiny of earlier assumptions, and texts are corrected to reflect such development. The process is further complicated by the vagaries of textual errors, not to mention the physical distress to which these perishable books are often subject.

Five such classical aggregations of ideas emerged some 2500 years ago as the primary sources of knowledge about Chinese culture and thought from what was then already China's ancient past. These are: *The Book of Changes (Yì Jīng); The Book of Songs (Shī Jīng); The Book of Rites (Lǐ Jì); The Book of History (Shū Jīng);* and *The Spring and Autumn Annals (Chūn Qiū).* To this day these are considered "The Five Classics" of the Chinese literary tradition. But this number comes nowhere near the number of literary works that have been collected during the past 2000 years. Medical classics alone number more than ten thousand. Thus all we can accomplish here is an introduction to the nature of the literary transmission through a brief examination of an important handful of ancient works.

 ## THE *YÌ JĪNG*—BOOK OF *CHANGES*

Any discussion of the literary tradition in China must begin with the *Yì Jīng.* The oldest of all the Chinese classics, its origin cannot be precisely dated. The earliest forms of the "text" of this ancient book of wisdom and prophecy consisted of inscriptions scratched into bones, often the broad shoulder bones of oxen. These "oracle bones" were part of the ancient tradition of magical intervention between two dimensions inhabited both by humans and by a variety of spiritual forces and entities thought to have varying degrees of influence on human affairs.

One interpretation of the origins of the *Yì Jīng* is that ancient necromancers heated the shells of turtles causing them to crack. Meaning was found in the shape and nature of the fissures. In time, from these patterns of cracks, a set of abstractions was codified to which various commentaries, images, explications, and advice were appended.

The traditional explanation of the Yì Jīng's origins describes an event in the life of the legendary "Emperor" of pre-historic China, Fu Xi. "Fu Xi listened to the eight winds," says the ancient story, "and, thus inspired, he set down the eight basic signs [from which the Yì Jīng is constructed]."

What is the Yì Jīng? Westerners have been trying to answer this question for several centuries now. The earliest Europeans to discover this ancient text were probably the Franciscan and Jesuit monks who first traveled to China. According to legend, more than one of these unfortunate clerics ended their lives in utter madness, their minds destroyed by something sinister and mysterious, long feared by the Chinese to exist within the ancient text of the Yì Jīng.

Like much of traditional Chinese culture, the image of the Yì Jīng is severely distorted when it appears in Western translations. The Yì Jīng arises from a primitive, prehistoric tradition of necromancy, geomancy, numerology, and word magic. It is the primary literary source of the theory of yīn and yáng. In its essence, the Yì Jīng is a mathematical schematic of the phenomenological universe of man and nature, heaven and earth.

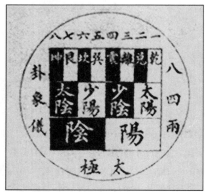

Chart showing the correspondence between tài jí, yīn-yáng, the four manifestations, and the eight basic trigrams of the Yì Jīng

This schematic is based upon a binary-like mathematical sequence that predates the binary notation of Leibniz by millennia. In fact, Leibniz had access to early Jesuit translations of the Yì Jīng. Joseph Needham mentions in the second volume of *Science and Civilization in China* that Leibniz conducted a protracted correspondence with the Jesuit missionary Joachim Bouvet mainly focused upon Bouvet's translations of the Yì Jīng and related materials. We cannot resist the speculation that this ancient Chinese material may have influenced the baroque German scholar.

In his own commentaries upon it, Leibniz wrote that the Yì Jīng was an ancient precursor of his concept of binary notation. Needham goes so far as to speculate that it was Fr. Bouvet who first suggested in a letter to Leibniz that the broken and unbroken lines of the Yì Jīng could be taken to represent the "0" and "1" of binary notation. Whatever the influence exerted on Leibniz in the course of his development and

WHO CAN RIDE THE DRAGON?

expression of this important aspect of mathematics in the West, the fact remains that thousands of years before it was developed in the West, a kind of binary mathematics flourished in prehistoric China as a medium for developing descriptors of phenomena.

We say "a kind of binary mathematics," because there are certainly fundamental differences between the mathematics of the Yì Jīng and pure binary notation. The gist of these differences lies in the fact that the mathematics of the Yì Jīng, though apparently formulated from a base-two system of reckoning, is actually formulated from a base-three notation. Its symbols are understood in terms of two sets of tripartate images: 1) the three realms of heaven, earth, and humankind; and 2) the relationship between yīn, yáng, and qì. These are the central relationships of Chinese thought.

From this viewpoint, the Yī Jīng describes the entire range of conditions that exist throughout the universe from which arise all natural phenomena. This is based upon a subset of eight basic structural components, the eight trigrams, which are attributed to the legendary Emperor, Fu Xi. The eight trigrams are themselves formed from the mathematically possible combinations of yīn and yáng within the three-fold context. This threefold context, represented as the three lines or places in each trigram, represents the three fundamental aspects of existence that concerned the ancient authors of the Yì Jīng: heaven, earth, and humanity. Implicit in this relationship is the relation of yīn, yáng, and qì.

The eight signs or "trigrams" represent eight essential images of the interaction between yīn and yáng. Each trigram consists of three lines or positions. There are two possible line types: one is yīn ; one is yáng. A yīn line is represented by a broken line, --. A yáng line is represented as an unbroken line, —. The basic form of the trigram is composed by assigning one line to stand for each of the three realms—earth, humankind, and heaven.

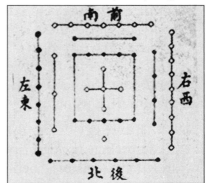

*River Chart of the eight trigrams,
said to derive from
a tattoo on the back of a horse
emerging from the Yellow River*

There are eight possible trigrams, the mathematical result of two-to-the-third power. The ancient Chinese observed a direct correspondence between these eight signs and the eight cardinal points (the eight "points" of the compass). For them, wind was the symbol of change that blew through the three realms carrying messages, energies, and influences—hence the legendary explanation that Fu Xi listened to the eight winds for inspiration.

Why? What do these eight simple glyphs represent? The logic is simple, eloquent, and comprehensive. It is embodied in a line from a later literary classic, the *Dào Dé Jīng:*

> *Dào gives birth to one.*
> *One gives birth to two.*
> *Two gives birth to three.*
> *Three gives birth to ten thousand things.*

China's ancient metaphysical mathematicians required only the first three prime numbers to evolve a descriptor of the entire universe and all phenomena contained therein. The *Dào,* which you recall from earlier discussions, comes from *wú jí* (infinity). It gives birth to heaven or yáng, the number of which is one. This one gives birth to earth or yīn, the number of which is two. Yīn and yáng give birth to *qì,* the number of which is three. And, *qì* gives birth to everything, the number of which is ten thousand. In Chinese, "ten thousand" symbolically means "numberless," hence "all."

One of the clearest statements than can be made about yīn and yáng is that everything comes from the interaction of yīn and yáng. When yīn and yáng unite, there is *qì,* thus there is life. When they separate, there is death. The interplay of yīn and yáng results in the unimaginable variety of objects and experience that we call existence. Therefore, we should be able to construct a comprehensive, if abstract, description of the universe using only yīn and yáng as the medium of description.

This was evidently the aim of ancients who developed precisely that: a comprehensive description of the universe using only yīn and yáng and their invisible coefficient, *qì.* The work of formulating the basic signs was attributed to the legendary Fu Xi. Perhaps they were the inspired effort of one superhuman, or maybe he found them on the back of a turtle or a horse (as variant versions of their legendary origins suggest). More likely they represent the gradual accumulation of insight and understanding over generations.

WHO CAN RIDE THE DRAGON?

These eight essential images could not in and of themselves be relied upon to provide the descriptions of phenomena that must have interested the ancient authors of the Yì Jīng. Things are, after all, not merely their essences. Things, objects, phenomena, and experiences are the manifestation of those essences. Thus, to express this manifest essence, the ancient Chinese created a set of doubled trigrams or "hexagrams" to be the basic functional unit of the mathematical language used to abstractly express all the possible changes that the world of man and nature experience as a result of the alternations of yīn and yáng.

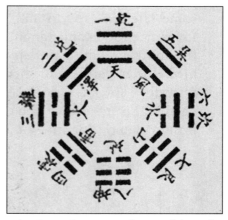

The classical correspondences of the eight trigrams with the points of the compass

The Yì Jīng is therefore an ancient digital "processor" that sought, in a way analogous to what hardware designers do today, to reduce phenomena to a mathematical grid and then construct functional patterns of "on" and "off" to relay information and instructions concerning the management of that information. This sort of operation in the hands of a competent, modern computer designer is aimed at developing things considered practical and important by cultural standards or demands. In a similar fashion, the goal of China's ancient sages was to codify experience and insight concerning the essential nature of things and their interrelations.

They sought to extend their knowledge to the utmost. To preserve the integrity of their work, and the power prediction provides, they encrypted it, much as contemporary encryption systems allow us to do today. They used a series of symbolic images which meant absolutely nothing until an initiate held the key that revealed their meaning.

To restate: the Yì Jīng is the fundamental treatise on yīn and yáng. It proposes, and many still believe achieves, a comprehensive description of phenomena based solely on the interaction of yīn and yáng. Although the gist of the theory of yīn and yáng developed in the works of the Daoists, its essential form comes directly from the Yì Jīng. As such, the importance of this most ancient Chinese classic in traditional Chinese medical theory cannot be overstated. If you ask a hundred doctors of Chinese medicine what they are doing when they treat their patients, you may well get a hundred different answers. But each one will contain some reference to yīn and yáng, even if it is not so explicitly stated. Reference to yīn and yáng is present (or certainly should be present) in the strategic thinking of any adequately trained practitioner of Chinese medicine, regardless of their specialization, regardless of their means, regardless of the formulas prescribed, or the points selected for needling. A traditional doctor of Chinese medicine is always working to bring yīn and yáng into a relatively more harmonious state.

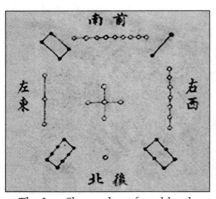

The Luo Shu, a chart found by the legendary Yu on the back of a tortoise in the Luo River. The nine places on the chart served as the basic pattern for dividing farm land, an essential blueprint of Chinese social structure.

This should not suggest that every doctor of Chinese medicine is a student of the Yì Jīng. Indeed, most of the Chinese doctors with whom we have spoken say frankly that their medical studies leave them no time for such esoteric pursuits. None-the-less, although it has always been shrouded in mystery and obscurity, the Yì Jīng has provided Chinese medicine, and Chinese civilization in general, with the essence of its internal coherence. As we have noted, the unique character of both yīn and yáng is that they are always changing. Change itself becomes the constant, all-pervasive internal coherence, and change is precisely the interplay and harmony of yīn and yáng.

Not only is this dynamism rooted philosophically, mathematically, and literally in the Yì Jīng, its life-sustaining currents circulate through the entire body of traditional medicial theory. In fact, there is an entire specialization in Chinese medicine which focuses on the direct relation-ships between the Yì Jīng and medicine.

Zhang Jie Bin of the Ming Dynasty composed a book entitled Lèi Jīng Fù Yì (Appended Wings of the Classified Classic), written in 1624 C.E. The first chapter, entitled "Medicine and Yì" contains the following explana-tion. (Yì is the Yì Jīng).

> Yì possesses the rationale of medicine. Medicine acquired the func-tion of the Yì. To only study medicine and not Yì leaves an impres-sion that medicine is not so difficult. And, indeed, it would be so. But who can know the sight of that which the eyes have yet to see? Who can know the sound of that which the ears have not yet heard?

WHO CAN RIDE THE DRAGON?

In the end, we cannot avoid the oneness of the composition of these two [the Yì Jīng and medicine]. For to know only the Yì and not medicine would lead one to say how difficult, mysterious, and vague the theories are; how hard they would be to put to use. It is no different than one who dreads the cold but refuses to wear a fur coat. It is the same as starving and refusing to eat the food one holds in one's own hand. What a pity to miss the opportunity of a lifetime! Thus medicine cannot proceed without the Yì. The Yì cannot proceed without medicine. The Sage Sun [Si Miao] said, "If one does not know the Yì, he is not qualified to discuss the Great Medicine."

If the rationale of heaven and earth is contained within the Yì, then how could the body and the mind not be contained by the Yì? Because of the motility of the Yì, because of its changes, the ancient model of anatomy in Chinese medicine is contained in the sixty-four hexagrams.

The application of the Yì Jīng to the theory and practice of medicine is an extraordinarily complex subject. Yet the relationship between the Yì Jīng and Chinese medicine can not be overlooked by those who wish to understand either subject thoroughly.

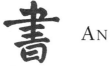 # ANCIENT MEDICAL CLASSICS

One of the most remarkable aspects of Chinese medicine is that the basic textbooks upon which virtually all others depend for their theoretical foundations are nearly 2000 years old. We have selected three of these ancient classics that represent the earliest extant codification of medical theories, principles of diagnosis and treatment, and the use of herbal medicines.

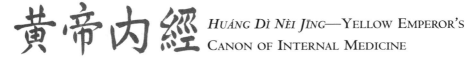 ## *HUÁNG DÌ NÈI JĪNG*—YELLOW EMPEROR'S CANON OF INTERNAL MEDICINE

This earliest medical work is written as a series of questions and answers. The legendary Yellow Emperor queries his Chief Physician, Qi Bo, on a wide range of issues concerning the nature of health and well-being, the method of attaining longevity, and the theory and practice of medicine. As with much Chinese classical literature, the authorship of this book is unknown. Without a doubt, it reflects the processes of literary transmission in ancient China that so profoundly shaped the form and content of ancient materials. Those who receive, study, transcribe, and transmit such material invariably add their own commentaries. They commit unwitting errors in transcription, delete material that seems unworthy of inclusion from their particular perspective, and so on.

An edition considered definitive was compiled by the Tang Dynasty physician Wang Bing in the eighth century and has served as the basis of subsequent versions. In fact, this process of constantly reshaping Chinese classical works continues today just as it has for millennia. This can be seen quite clearly in how the *Yellow Emperor's Canon* has come to be understood outside of China.

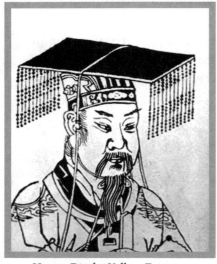

Huang Di–the Yellow Emperor

The book that is traditionally understood to be the *Huáng Dì Nèi Jīng (Yellow Emperor's Internal Canon)* consists of two main parts. The first is called *Sù Wèn* or *Simple Questions*. The second is called *Líng Shū* or *Miraculous Spiritual Pivot* and is largely devoted to the theory and practice of acupuncture. For many years in the West, there was but one major translation of the book, done by the sinologist/sociologist Ilza Veith. Regrettably, her translation included only the *Sù Wèn* portion of the text—only one-fifth, more or less, of the classical text—an omission that has left many Western readers with the impression that this one-fifth is the complete work.

Thus the literary tradition, subjected to the vagaries of translation, has suffered in transmission; and the complexity and difficulty associated with conscientious study is compounded.

The problem is analogous to the trade in ancient Chinese artifacts such as ceramics, paintings, and other works of art. Copying and forging works of art is an occupation that has flourished in China for thousands of years. The people of one period, favoring the works of a particular prior epoch, collected artifacts from that time with which to ornament their homes. When the supplies of a particular period ran low, or

WHO CAN RIDE THE DRAGON?

when demand forced prices high, craftsmen seized the opportunity to provide eager buyers with ingeniously forged copies. Thus, it is possible today to find Ming Dynasty forgeries of Tang Dynasty ceramics. The quality of scholarship and expert sensitivity required to properly sort such work is amazing.

It is important to perceive the contents of a book such as *The Yellow Emperor's Canon* in the rich and complicated matrix of culture, art, and science from which it arose. One awareness we develop studying these traditions is that things are seldom what they may seem to Western eyes. This literary tradition contains a strong predilection towards letting subtle and complex material emerge slowly from the interaction of student and teacher. The books themselves were never meant to stand alone in the way we think of modern textbooks. Traditionally, the transmission of medical arts and sciences in China consisted not just of studying the ancient texts but of having them illuminated by a teacher who had been similarly enlightened.

Thus when we look at the *Yellow Emperor's Canon of Internal Medicine* we should understand that it is an early blueprint of Chinese medicine. It contains the main theoretical elements. It describes the ways in which these elements interrelate. It provides definitions for basic terminology. The word *qì*, for example, is used with some 270 different meanings in this one book alone.

The *Huáng Dì Nèi Jīng* defines disease, and more importantly it contains a comprehensive definition of health. It asserts the fundamental strategy that a student and practitioner of the medical arts must follow to benefit from the wisdom of China's ancient sages. In this regard it is important to stress again another basic issue already mentioned earlier. This is the spiritual or philosophical dimension of Chinese medicine. One of the things that clearly distinguishes traditional medicine in China from the modern scientific and technological medicine of the West is this spiritual dimension. Chinese medicine differs in a fundamental way from Western medicine that can be summarized thus: since its earliest origins, Chinese medicine has focused intensively on the spiritual, emotional, psychological, and philosophical aspects of disease and wellbeing.

The roots of such concerns are found in the *Yellow Emperor's Canon*. The implications for contemporary healthcare professionals are considerable, for from this broad and comprehensive approach to medical theory a uniquely Chinese strategy of preventive medicine emerges. The passage mentioned in Chapter 3 contains the gist of this strategy:

> The ancient sages did not treat those who had already become ill; they did not try to rule those who were already rebellious. Instead, they preferred to educate the people before they rebelled. They treated their patients before they could get sick. Treating people who are sick with herbs and acupuncture can be compared to the behavior of people who only start forging their weapons after they are engaged in battle or to those who only think of digging a well after they feel thirsty. Aren't such actions just a little late?

難經 NÁN JĪNG—THE CLASSIC OF DIFFICULT ISSUES

Originally called *The Classic of Eighty-One Difficulties,* this book, like the *Yellow Emperor's Canon,* is of uncertain origin. It resembles the *Yellow Emperor's Canon* in an important way: both are written as dialogues. Additionally, both books were probably compiled in the first or second century B.C.E., the *Yellow Emperor's Canon* likely being somewhat earlier.

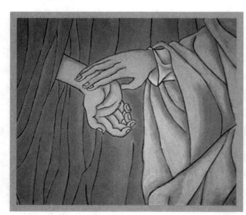

Detail of a painting showing pulse diagnosis

The eighty-one questions that comprise the text of the *Nán Jīng* are divided into several categories. Questions one through twenty-two deal with the subject of pulse diagnosis. This subject was illuminated in this series of questions and answers for the first time. Here we find the definitions of the three positions for taking the pulse: *cùn, guān, and chǐ,* each on the radial artery at the wrist. Based on this early material, pulse diagnosis later developed into a fundamental skill of medicine in China.

Questions twenty-three through twenty-nine concern the study of the *jīng luò* or channels and network vessels through which the *qì* circulates throughout the entire body. Questions thirty through forty-seven deal with the internal organs, their structure, function, and interrelationships. From question forty-eight through sixty-one the subject of inquiry is illness and the processes leading to disease. Questions sixty-two through

WHO CAN RIDE THE DRAGON?

sixty-eight discuss the location and function of acupuncture points, and questions sixty-nine through eighty-one deal with acupuncture theory and techniques. Thus the *Nán Jīng* is a comprehensive outline of basic medical theory, internal medicine, and acupuncture treatment.

This book also develops the theories of the *mìng mén* or "gate of life" and the "triple burner" or *sān jiāo* that are found in the *Yellow Emperor's Canon*. This early codification of medical theory and principles of treatment contributed greatly to the development of medicine in later eras, making the *Nán Jīng* an indispensable classic of traditional Chinese medicine.

傷 寒 論 *Shāng Hán Lùn*—On Cold Damage

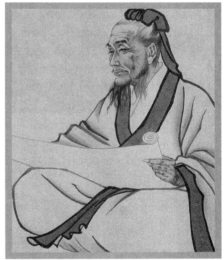

This work was originally entitled *Treatise on Cold Damage and Miscellaneous Diseases*. Unlike the two works discussed above, its origin has long been established with virtual certainty. Its author was one of China's most famous doctors, Zhang Zhong Jing, who lived in the Eastern Han period (25–220 C.E.). The book's influence on the development of medicine in China and throughout East Asia has been profound. Today there are entire departments in colleges and universities of traditional medicine in China devoted to the study of this single work.

Portrait of Zhang Zhong Jing, courtesy Lifu Museum, China Medical College, Taiwan

The preface of the book states that there are sixteen volumes, but this conflicts with the number known to exist. For some eight centuries, the book was handed down as a single composition, but in the Song Dynasty, it was subjected to the same process of reexamination and correction that was applied to a wide range of intellectual and academic disciplines at that time. The "Imperial Bureau of Rectifying Medical Texts" issued a revised and corrected version which separated material from the original book into two parts. One was entitled *Essential Prescriptions from the Golden Cabinet;* the other was called *Treatise on Damage from Cold*. Even today this remains the organization of the material that has survived.

The work systematized the study of clinical medicine, establishing and defining the basic principles of diagnosis and treatment through the identification and differentiation of patterns of disease. It also presented hundreds of formulas of herbal medicine along with the indications for their use. To this day, these formulas comprise the backbone of traditional Chinese pharmaceutics. They are so highly respected throughout the Orient that in Japan, for example, only those herbal prescriptions based on formulas from the *Shāng Hán Lùn* will be reimbursed by health insurance.

Zhang Zhong Jing is revered as the "Sage of Medicine." His book is known as the "book that brings people life." Generally, in Chinese the term "classical formula" is reserved to refer to formulas he composed. He is indisputably one of the greatest theorists of traditional Chinese medicine. His theoretical contributions include not only the specification of cold damage and the effect of external influences on human health, but also the design of a disease progression theory that has influenced traditional Chinese medicine until today. Although the *Shāng Hán Lùn* "six-channel pattern identification" theory Zhang Zhong Jing refined from the *Inner Canon (Nèi Jīng)* would be constantly adapted, particularly by the later text *Wēn Bìng (Warm Disease)*, the theory, its diagnostic indications, and treatment patterns are one of the mainstays of traditional practice.

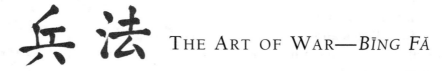 THE ART OF WAR—*BĪNG FǍ*

The *Art of War* is one of the world's classic treatises on strategy and warfare. The author, Sun Zi, was a general of the State of Qi during the Period of Spring and Autumn (770–476 B.C.E.). The principles of military strategy contained in this book have informed the Chinese military ever since, and is widely studied in military academies around the world.

Recently, this Chinese classic has become popular in the United States. Corporate executives study it. One Hollywood mogul was rumored to have made it required reading for his entire staff. The book has found such widespread acceptance as a source of strategic wisdom that it could rightfully be called a contemporary classic as well as an ancient one. Perhaps Western business people, recognizing that sooner or later they would find themselves in competition with their Asian contemporaries, have taken up the *Art of War* to prepare themselves for inevitable confrontations. Perhaps, noticing the remarkable success of the overseas Chinese in a wide variety of commercial ventures and the staggering economic expansion currently underway on the Chinese mainland, Western readers seek to educate themselves in what may well be a superior approach to strategic thinking.

Regardless of what motivates these thousands of Western readers, the most important thing to note is the value Chinese thinkers place on strategic thinking and a well-conceived and logical plan of action. This is the central lesson for those who embrace Sun Zi's *Art of War*. As a landmark in Chinese cultural history, the *Art of War* clearly indicates the importance of strategy for those who have recorded and transmitted the Chinese legacy from generation to generation.

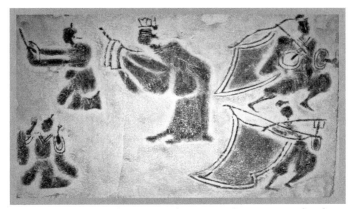

Rubbing from a Han dynasty tomb carving, depicting ritualized gestures employed on the battlefield which illustrate Sun Zi's Art of War

To Chinese thinkers, the ability to assess situations and make practical, successful strategic decisions looms large. It is not therefore solely racial stereotyping, or ill-spirited racism, when people around the world describe the Chinese as "crafty" or "inscrutable." The Chinese people possess and prize a tradition of cunning, as reflected in the first of Sun Zi's thirty-six stratagems that epitomize traditional Chinese strategic thinking: "No deception is too great." The *Art of War* serves as an important vessel for this tradition, and it should be well studied and understood by any who seek to understand traditional Chinese culture and its various artifacts.

It may be less apparent, but this same approach to strategic thinking informs much of traditional Chinese medicine. The roots of the logic that express as treatment principles, herbal formulas, and acupoint prescriptions grow in a soil fertilized by the *Art of War*. Thus its study in the context of Chinese medicine is not merely an interesting sidelight, but a beacon that illuminates the underlying intellectual mechanisms of medical theories and techniques. Many doctors of Chinese medicine conceive of medical intervention as a war between the "righteous *qì*" (*zhèng qì*) and the "evil *qì*" (*xié qì*). This is reflected in a number of Chinese medical terms.

For example, the aspect of *qì* that relates to the body's protective mechanisms (functions generally ascribed to the immune system in biomedical thought) is termed "defense *qì*" or *wèi qì* in Chinese medicine. The Chinese word *wèi* comes directly from military parlance where it refers to the guards who stand at the perimeter of an army's encampment to defend against invaders. A complementary concept, again reflecting this martial sensibility, is contained in yet another aspect of *qì*: *yíng qì*. The word *yíng* originally meant "camp" or "construction" (in the sense of setting up an army camp). The *yíng qì* is the aspect of the *qì* that circulates the nourishment derived from food throughout the body so that it can be used to construct new tissue and repair organs, flesh, and sinew. In terms of this martial metaphor, it is the *yíng* encampment of the body that is defended by the *wèi* guards.

This martial metaphor can be seen in the use of another important pair of medical terms, *xū* and *shí*. These terms have been given many English equivalents, including empty and full; insubstantial and substantial; deplete and replete; vacuous and replete; deficient and excess. In Chinese medicine these are the key terms used to describe the complementary and contrasting conditions from which disease processes and disharmonies result. Thus, if acupuncture points are found to be *xū* or vacuous, a doctor will treat them with a supplementing technique, to fill the vacuity. If a point is pathologically *shí* or replete, it must be drained to draw off the damaging or blocking *qì* that it has accumulated. Diseases are likewise categorized according to their prevailing characteristics in terms of *xū* and *shí*. It is this differentiation which allows a doctor to prescribe herbal formulas to supplement what is *xū* and drain what is *shí*.

In the following passages taken from the *Art of War,* we see that before vacuity, *xū* 虛, and repletion, *shí* 實, were employed as medical terms, Sun Zi used them to describe principles governing the conduct of military maneuvers. In Chapter Five, Sun Zi says:

> *The arrangement of military attacks is like throwing a stone at an egg. The key lies in xū and shí.*

He elaborates in Chapter Six:

> *Thus military force is like water. The movement of water always avoids the high places and tends towards the low. The deployment of military force avoids the shí to attack the xū, following directions to accord with the physical features of the place [of battle]. The victory of the military accords with [conditions of] the enemy. Thus the army does not have a fixed method of deploying its forces just as water has no fixed shape. If the changes of the enemy are ascertained and lead to victory, it is called mysterious [literally shén— spirit, mystery, marvel]. Thus the five phases have no fixed order of restraint. The four seasons have no fixed position. The day's length appears long or short. The moon waxes and wanes.*

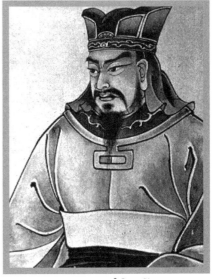

Portrait of Sun Zi

Here Sun Zi is probably referring to a concept of ancient Chinese lunar astronomy describing 28 constellations separated into four groups according to the four seasons. The formulation of the ancient calendar depended upon this system of reckoning to determine the appearance of the night sky in each season. Due to the nature of this ancient Chinese lunar calendar, the position of these constellations appears to change slightly from year to year.

Sun Zi also relied on the concept of *qì* to describe principles of how to gain military victory. In Chapter Seven he states:

> *Even the qì of numerous troops can be captured if the heart of the commander can be captured. The qì of morning dashes out. The qì of midday is indolent. At dusk the qì is exhausted. One who is adept in the use of military force avoids the dashing qì and attacks when*

it is indolent or exhausted. Thus he controls the qì. Use order to treat
chaos. Use tranquility to treat an uproar. Thus, control the heart.

It is more than a coincidence that the language at the end of this passage sounds almost as if Sun Zi is describing medical concepts. Compare,
for example, the following passage from "The Great Treatise on the
Manifestations of Yīn and Yáng" in the *Yellow Emperor's Canon of Internal
Medicine:*

> *Thus, in diseases of the yáng, treat the yīn. In diseases of the yīn,*
> *treat the yáng.*

This is only one example among a vast number that can be cited to
demonstrate the internal coherence that develops from the theory of yīn
and yáng. This internal coherence binds the theory and practice of medicine together with a wide range of philosophical, literary and cultural
phenomena. In fact what appears from outside the Chinese cultural
milieu as separate subjects—military strategy, philosophy, medicine,
and art—can be considered as distinct manifestations of a single paradigm when viewed from within.

From the clinical point of view, a curious fact about Chinese medicine is that ten different clinicians may devise ten different treatment
principles for the same patient. When we interview these ten practitioners, however, we find that each employs a sense of strategic thinking in
arriving at his or her conclusions and that the gist of the principles of
strategy thus employed will often have origins in the *Art of War.*

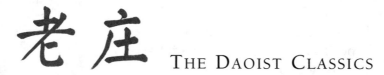 THE DAOIST CLASSICS

There is much lively debate among academicians concerning the identity of the authors, editors, and creators of the key works of Daoism. Who
came first, Zhuang or Lao? Which *Dào* is the real *Dào*? Such questions,
if satisfactorily answered, may have an enormous influence upon our
reading and understanding of Daoist texts. They are, however, as yet
both unknown and not necessarily germane to understanding Chinese
medicine. In the simple view, there is a common understanding of the
two texts that most exemplify the Daoist literary tradition. It is a tradition that is rich and complicated, despite the absolute simplicity of its

most fundamental precepts. The *Dào Dé Jīng,* attributed to the legendary Lao Zi, is the cornerstone of Daoist thought. But beneath this cornerstone lies a single word which forms the most important cognitive artifact of this unique philosophical and literary tradition.

The Chinese word *dào* contains a powerful metaphor from which countless meanings have arisen. In its simple, literal sense, the word means "road." In contemporary Chinese it is used to identify streets of a certain size, capacity, or characteristic. In much the same manner as the English words, "boulevard," "avenue," "street", "lane," and "way," Chinese words like *dào, jiē,* and *lù,* categorize the streets of a Chinese city by their varying widths, lengths, capacities, and ambiance. The word "*dào*" also has other modern meanings more closely related to its ancient sense and philosophical use. This metaphoric usage derives from the juxtaposition of the elements of the word itself.

Since ancient times, the word symbolized a way of seeing, thinking about, and living in the world. "Awareness in motion" or "the way you go as a result of thinking," are somewhat awkward English-language phrases that nevertheless convey the essential nature of this character. (See p. 81 for a further discussion of its meaning.) Considered as such, the word "*dào*" expresses an important precept of Daoist thought which is seldom mentioned in the texts themselves; indeed in Zhuang Zi there is no direct mention of it. This precept is the notion that the world and everything in it is essentially a work of the imagination, a product of the mind as it moves along.

This *dào* of Zhuang Zi characterizes perhaps the best known of Zhuang Zi's fables. It is the story of himself, dreaming he is a butterfly. When he awakens, he experiences a typically Daoist paradox concerning the nature of reality. He doesn't know, in that moment poised between waking and dreaming, whether he is Zhuang Zi waking from a dream of being a butterfly, or if he is a butterfly dreaming of being Zhuang Zi.

The character *dào* contains this dimension of meaning, that is, the central role of the process of consciousness in the nature of "reality." To understand the multidimensional outlook of the Daoists, we must look further into the literary roots of the subject. The literature of Chinese traditional subjects can be understood like a series of postcards from ancient correspondents. In order to streamline their messages to future generations, these ancient custodians of wisdom condensed their understanding into as few strokes as possible.

The kernels of their wisdom thus lie waiting in the words themselves. These Daoist texts have been preserved for nearly 2500 years. The precepts and concepts they convey are alive today in the theories of Chinese medicine.

道 德 經 THE *DÀO DÉ JĪNG*

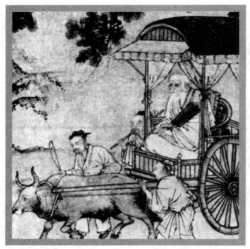

Detail from a hanging scroll by Shang Hsi, "Lao-tzu Passing the Barrier"

The *Dào Dé Jīng* (*Classic of the Way and Moral Virtue*) has a unique position in the literary tradition of ancient China. None can deny the power and influence that this book has had both within China and around the world. It presents and defines a concept that is extraordinarily difficult to catch hold of.

Confucius is reported to have said, after his first and only meeting with the legendary author of the *Dào Dé Jīng*, "Lao Zi is like a dragon!" In the introduction to his explications of Lao Zi, the great *Tài jí* master Zheng Man Qing succinctly states:

Although Lao-tzu [Lao Zi] was a profoundly practical man, human emotions disgusted him greatly, and he longed to get away. He hoped for a new beginning though metamorphosis, or, as the phrase has it, "his step leaves no footprint." How much more difficult it is to find the tracks of Lao-tzu's mind! Only one man understood, and that was Confucius. Did he not say Lao-tzu was like a dragon? How right he was! How can any flying or walking creature compare with dragon-like Lao-tzu?

The *Dào Dé Jīng* contains the essence of a philosophical system that grows from two indigenous Chinese sources. The first is a naturalistic metaphysics that deposits the source of all things, all energies, all actions in "limitless-ness" or *wú jí* and "non-action" or *wú wéi*. The second influence is an epistemology and cosmology deeply rooted in the ancient Chinese concept of yīn and yáng. The "dào" of Lao Zi is a shadowy thing from which arise all phenomena in the universe. The Sage's advice in the presence of such knowledge is to relax, give up all strenuous effort, and follow the natural timing of change.

For most it is a philosophy which simply defies adherence. Many rant against it as a source of indolence and sloth, although these are hardly virtues that could have survived through the esteem of a community that struggled to eke its survival from the land. Yet despite what has been characterized at times as a despicable impracticality, this philosophy of following the natural way has persisted as a constant thread in the tapestry of life in China.

Chapter 48 of the 81 brief chapters that comprise the traditional classic gives poignant advice as to how to pursue this way of thinking and living:

> To pursue learning, accumulate day after day. To pursue the Dào, day after day you must lose. Lose and lose until you reach non-action. Non-action but nothing left undone. To gain mastery of the world you must get to the point of no undertakings. If motivated for gain, once you begin to act you won't get anywhere.

The book is full of similar admonitions. Although its esoteric philosophy presents considerable difficulties to those who seek to follow the Dào, in the two thousand years since its composition, more than fourteen hundred writers have offered interpretations of it.

The text itself reflects the paradoxical nature of a philosophy that seeks to harmonize human consciousness and human action with the great Dào of nature. Its images and meanings are alternately concrete and ethereal. One of the themes or motifs that winds through this puzzling labyrinth of poetic passageways is the "Mysterious Female, Mother of All Things." Chapter One says:

> What has no name is the origin of heaven and earth;
> what has a name is the Mother of all things.

The White Cloud Daoist temple in Beijing is the site of a shrine to this Mother of all things. It is situated in the centermost room of what may well be Daoism's most sacred place. Above the threshold there is an inscription to this Mother. Inside, the room is absolutely empty. Lao Zi makes constant reference to this notion of emptiness, this Mysterious Female as the source of all things. In Chapter Six he wrote:

The spirit of the valley does not die, and is called Mysterious Female.
The door of the Mysterious Female is called the root of heaven and
earth.

In Chapter Four we read:

The Dào is empty, yet when used is never filled up. So deep it seems
to be the ancestor of all things.

Lao Zi wrote of the "indescribable marvels" which could be achieved by conforming to the principles and movement of the Dào. The method he advised was itself, like its subject, "shadowy and indistinct." In Chapter Three, Lao Zi provided some concrete instructions to those who would seek to follow his subtle and esoteric path:

The Sage governs himself by relaxing the mind, reinforcing the
abdomen, gentling the will, strengthening the bones.

Tài jí quán, developed in the Song Dynasty as a method of self-defense and personal cultivation through the principles of Daoism, conforms to this advice and stands as an ideal illustration of ways in which successive generations of Chinese philosophers sought to interpret and apply their understanding of Lao Zi. In the slow-moving and relaxed postures of the solo exercises of *tài jí*, one sees the Daoist principles embodied and animated in the movements. Later authors, inspired by their Daoist ancestors, wrote that *tài jí* is like a great river, rolling on unceasingly.

In such remarks they evoked an image that flows everywhere through the *Dào Dé Jīng*: the image of water. For Lao Zi, water was like the highest good. In water's complete non-resistance to the forces it encounters, Lao Zi found the ideal metaphor for the movement of the Dào.

Water is a positive benefit to all things without competing with them.
It seeks out places abominated by man. Thereby, it approaches the
Dào.

Using this metaphor of water as his standard, Lao Zi advised readers to "attain utmost emptiness. Maintain profound tranquillity." Only thus could earthly affairs be brought into a state of balance and equilibrium. It is this attitude which gave rise to the statement that governing a great nation was like "cooking a small fish." The message is remarkably similar to the political philosophy of Thomas Jefferson, who said, "That government which governs least, governs best."

In Chapter Sixteen of the *Dào Dé Jīng,* Lao Zi emphasized keeping to the roots of primitive naturalistic philosophy that run deep throughout Daoism and into traditional medical theory:

> *All things are stirring about. I watch their cycle. Things flourish and each returns to its root. This is what is meant by returning to one's basic nature. Returning to one's basic nature is called constancy. To understand constancy is called enlightening. Not to understand constancy is to blindly do unfortunate things.*

This way of thinking and of expressing thoughts has had a profound influence on the development of culture in China. Though it has never actually been embraced and utilized as a blueprint for governing the country, the *Dào* of Lao Zi has insinuated itself into virtually every aspect of traditional Chinese culture.

Medicine benefited immeasurably from the influence of Lao Zi's enigmatic philosophy. Doctors of Chinese medicine come to understand their patients as puzzles or riddles, best understood and remedied through the comprehension of the specific imbalances of yīn and yáng that each individual patient presents. This is but a part of the legacy of Lao Zi, China's quintessential Old Man. It has served to quicken the perception, animate the imagination, and deepen the understanding of medical theorists for over 2000 years.

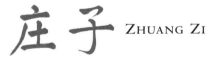 ZHUANG ZI

In contrast to the esoteric magic of Lao Zi, the second essential text of Daoism uses earthy parables to illustrate principles of Daoist thought. This text is known by the name of its author, Zhuang Zi. His whole name is Zhuang Zhou, and, according to oft-repeated legend, he lived in the Warring States Period, two or three hundred years after Lao Zi.

Like Lao Zi, Zhuang Zi preferred non-action. He has always been viewed as the paragon of high moral character and purity of spirit. One story illustrates these qualities well.

> *One day Zhuang Zi was fishing in the Pu River which runs through what is now Henan Province. The king of the state of Chu sent two emissaries to convey a message to the sage.*

"The King sends his regards," began the officials, when the came upon Zhuang Zi beside the river. "He instructs us to inform you that he entrusts you with the affairs of state and recognizes the bitter work that awaits you."

Without so much as turning his head, Zhuang Zi replied, "I have heard there is a divine tortoise in Chu which has been dead for 3000 years. I heard the king put it in a bamboo basket and covered it with silk. It sits, so I've been told, in the position of great esteem within the temple. But I wonder whether this divine tortoise would rather have its shell and bones become treasure or still be dragging its tail through the muddy water."

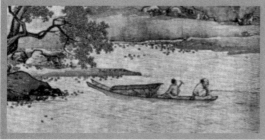

The two officials answered with a chuckle, "Of course, it would rather still be alive, dragging its tail through the mud!"

Zhuang Zi held his fishing rod still. "You'd better go now. For I, too, prefer to drag my tail through the mud."

"Secluded Fishermen on an Autumn River," T'ang Yin

In stories like this, Zhuang Zi communicated a body of concepts that came to have profound influence on Chinese thought. This way of thinking pervades the work of medical theorists. At the center of this body of concepts is the notion of the *Dào*. In Zhuang Zi, the concepts of *Dào* and *qì* are closely interlinked. In *Zhī Běi Yóu (Traveling to the North)*, he wrote, "The whole world is just *qì*."

> *Living is the gathering of qì. Death is the separation of qì. Life is the companion of death. Death is the beginning of life. Who can know where the beginning is? Who can know the rule?*

Such remarks contributed heavily to the skeptical mysticism of Daoism.

The subtle machinations of *qì*, taken together, comprise the *Dào*. This concept of the universality of *qì* as characterized in the *Zhuang Zi* became a cornerstone in the foundation of Chinese medical theory where it was further refined and developed. Certainly it is the most important point of view in diagnostics. This sense of *qì* as the medium for the interconnections of the universe and all of its phenomena provided Chinese medical theorists with an ideal model for explaining the relationships between individuals and the environmental factors that

WHO CAN RIDE THE DRAGON?

result in disease. In fact, it served as the typical explanation of the wholeness of the patient's body, mind, and spirit as well as their complex interrelationships with the environment. The *qì* of nature was seen to move through its changes in the natural world, and these movements were understood to influence the body, the mind, the spirit, and the whole state of being through processes understood as seamless extensions of environmental phenomena.

This is reflected in the terminology of Chinese medicine, as we will discuss in greater detail in Chapter 7. One clear example of this understanding is the names given acupoints. Acupuncture points were named after springs, hills, and valleys, in an analogy between *qì* and the water and wind that flowed through the "external" world. Zhuang Zi set forth the philosophical antecedent of this correlative thinking.

Another important concept from Zhuang Zi is the notion that everything is in a constant state of change and development. "There is no movement that does not change. No time fails to move on." This fundamental concept also found its way into many aspects of Chinese medical theory—for example, in the theory of disease transmission between various "levels" of the body. Thus, in Chinese diagnostics, the patient's presenting symptoms are not indicative of a fixed entity but of a stage within a shifting picture of disease. By clearly identifying the active stage and correctly correlating it with the appropriate theoretical pattern of change and progression from one stage to the next, the traditional doctor can treat not merely the present symptoms but can take effective steps against a likely future progression.

In other words, according to the most fundamental advice of the *Yellow Emperor's Canon,* a well-trained doctor of Chinese medicine can treat patients before they become more seriously ill. For the development of such subtle skills, doctors, even today, owe a debt of gratitude to the ancient sage, Zhuang Zi, whose whole attitude can be summed in one phrase: "Follow nature."

Like Lao Zi, Zhuang Zi placed a high value on the ability to quiet the will and seek repose in non-action.

> *Content in nothingness, non-action; holding the same position as heaven and earth: this is true virtue. Follow the middle way of nature as law. This can protect one's self, one's nature. This way one can enjoy and prolong life.*

An interesting point relating this saying of Zhuang Zi with Chinese medicine is that the word meaning "middle way" is the same word used to name the circulatory *qì* pathway or *jīng luò* of the *dū* channel, the extraordinary vessel channel that runs up the spine. This *dū* channel is the meeting point of all the *yáng qì* in the body. It commands or governs the movement and activity of the *yáng qì* of the whole body, just as Zhuang Zi suggests the "middle way" can take control of one's life and make it enjoyable and long. It becomes clear from such examples that the aims of medicine are closely linked to the aims of philosophers like Zhuang Zi and his followers.

Again, the philosophical orientation of traditional medicine in China is one of its distinguishing characteristics. To proceed into clinical practice, therefore, without a thorough grasp of the philosophical roots of traditional medical theories is not simply ill-advised; it constitutes a significant disservice to patients. For Chinese medicine is far more than a series of clinical techniques. It is a comprehensive system of logically derived interventions designed to foster, restore, and otherwise enhance the balance between the individual and the environment. Without access to this logic, the interventions lose their meaning and their efficacy. Without understanding the nature of its Daoist influences, the logic of Chinese medicine would be virtually impossible to grasp.

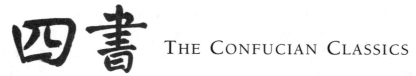 THE CONFUCIAN CLASSICS

Often referred to as "The Four Books," the classical books attributed to Confucius stand as cornerstones in the foundation of Chinese philosophy. The four books are *Dà Xué, Zhōng Yōng, Mèng Zǐ,* and *Lùn Yǔ.* The ideas and language contained in these books have had a profound influence on life in China for 2000 years. Even Chinese people who have never read them are conversant with many of their themes. They play a role in the coursework of every Chinese university student that is comparable to but even more intense and dramatic than how Western students study Thomas Paine, Karl Marx, or Plato. If anything, their influence in China is even more widespread than that of their Western counterparts. Indeed, after they were edited and revised by the Song Dynasty scholar Zhu Xi, the Confucian classics served as the basis of the Imperial civil service examination. Thus, for the next 700 years, virtually every Chinese civil servant had to prove his knowledge of these books to achieve an official position.

Nor did the importance of these books stop with officialdom. For countless generations, the Confucian tradition has symbolized Chinese thought and attitudes. Even the core of Chinese family and community life reflected the influence of these Confucian texts.

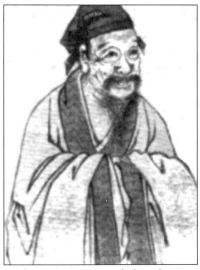

Since the earliest days of contact and exchange between China and the Western world, the contents of these Confucian texts have been translated, both poorly and exceedingly well, and have filled everything from the pages of lofty sinology journals to fortune cookies. The history and interpretation of these texts is so long and complicated that it serves as the subject for doctoral dissertations for those who wish to devote lifelong study to this quintessentially Chinese tradition of wisdom.

The Song Dynasty scholar Zhu Xi

We present the barest introduction to the works known as *Dà Xué* (*The Great Learning*) and *Zhōng Yōng* (*The Doctrine of the Mean*). Our selection of these two in no way implies that the other books are less significant. Neither should readers satisfy themselves with only our commentaries. We hope only to emphasize the enormous importance of the Confucian classics and stimulate you to investigate them more fully.

The rationale for focusing on these two works is that Confucian doctrine contains an important and sometimes overlooked idea. In his introduction to his translation of *Zhōng Yōng,* Ezra Pound pointed out that "the second of the Four Classics, *Chung Yung* [a variant romanization of *Zhōng Yōng*], the *Unwobbling Pivot,* contains what is usually supposed not to exist, namely the Confucian metaphysics." He went on to characterize it thus: "Only the most absolute sincerity under heaven can effect change."

There is a constant theme in both texts of "rectifying the heart" as the fundamental act of bringing oneself and one's actions into harmony with the "right way." Thus we come to know the *dào* of Confucius clearly through *Zhōng Yōng*. It is a way of thinking that permeates the Chinese mind, reflecting the central importance given to balance, harmony, and reserve in virtually every aspect of human behavior. It also exemplifies the attitude of humility with which a well-trained doctor of Chinese medicine approaches his or her study and practice.

The reason for focusing on *Dà Xué, The Great Learning,* is that it contains a virtual blueprint for the Confucian ideal of rectifying the heart, through the process of "precise verbal definitions of its inarticulate thoughts," leading to the ability to penetrate the deepest mysteries of existence. The influence of such a process is then delineated as the text instructs us how a well-ordered household and family life serves as the basis of order in the State and in good government.

This systematic sense of organized harmony developing from the ability to completely grasp the essence of things is a critical element in Chinese medical theory and application. There is no clearer iteration of the principles upon which such sensibilities are based than these two Confucian texts.

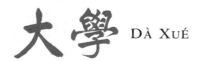 DÀ XUÉ

The Great Learning, as it is frequently translated into English, is one of the most studied of the Confucian classics. Like so much of the classical literature of China, this treatise on the relationship between acquiring knowledge (particularly of one's innermost nature) and the pursuit of harmonious conduct within family and social institutions can be interpreted in many different ways.

In his translation as well as his illumination of the text, Ezra Pound developed an English-language version which excels in bringing the spirit of the original to non-Chinese readers. We have consulted a number of Chinese scholars, and the general consensus we encountered is that Pound's interpretation of the text is not only basically sound, but poetically accurate. He provides an English version that has a hint of the original's flavor. Pound's translation focuses intently upon the deeper meanings of the individual characters. In short, his work of translating the text becomes an extension of the work itself in the finest sense of a Chinese literary classic. The Confucian text urges that one engage in the process leading to "precise verbal definitions," and Pound responded by doing precisely that. This can be seen clearly in the following passage.

> The men of old, wanting to clarify and diffuse throughout the empire that light which comes from looking straight into the heart and then acting, first set up good government in their own states; wanting good government in their states, they first established order in their own families; wanting order in the home, they first disciplined themselves; desiring self-discipline, they rectified their own hearts; and wanting to rectify their hearts, they sought precise verbal definitions of their inarticulate thoughts [the tones given off by the heart]; wishing to attain precise verbal definitions, they set to extend their knowledge to the utmost. This completion of knowledge is rooted in sorting things into organic categories.

There are many things that could be said about this passage. For instance, one sees reflected in it an important piece of traditional anatomical understanding. In Pound's parenthetical note (set off in brackets above) he points out the literal definition of "thoughts" in the Chinese text. In the phrase, "the tones given off by the heart" we can quite clearly see how ancient Chinese conceived of the heart as the seat of consciousness. This same sensibility appears in traditional Chinese diagnostic terminology for certain mental disorders. "Phlegm confounding the orifices of the heart" is a phrase that describes a category of mental illness characterized by various, relatively mild symptoms and symptomatic patterns of behavior. It is, however, an altogether different diagnosis when liver fire rises to harass the heart and more virulent symptoms appear.

One of the identifying characteristics of Chinese medical theory is its comprehensive approach to the body as an integrated whole. Ancient anatomists and physiologists were more concerned with the overall function of the living organism than with a detailed description of the material dimension of being human. They beheld a dynamic system of interdependent mechanisms, functions, structures, and substances and sought to evolve a method for intervening when disease and dysfunction occurred. More importantly, they were guided by ancient advice to treat their patients before they became ill, to prevent rather than to treat disease.

This sort of strategic thinking relates directly to the passage quoted above from the Dà Xué, as it does to several other Chinese classics discussed in this chapter. The selection of a treatment principle in Chinese medicine can also be understood as an exercise in strategy similar to that employed on the field of battle. Alternately, medical intervention can be understood as the governance of the empire of the body. These two metaphors, at less variance in the ancient feudal world than they may seem today, are fundamentally aligned in their conception of the body in terms of natural, social, and military structures which must be wisely managed in order to maintain the harmony of yīn and yáng, *qì* and blood, *jīng* and *shén*.

In *Dà Xué,* Confucius presents a method or formula for placing a whole nation in a state of harmony and balance. This formula, relying on intimate self-knowledge—listening to the tones given off by one's heart—is also perfectly applicable to the managment of medical intervention. It has indeed informed the thinking of Chinese medical experts for centuries. This subject is developed in even greater detail in another of the Confucian classics, *Zhōng Yōng* (*The Unwobbling Pivot,* as Pound termed it).

The whole Confucian strategy is aimed at self-cultivation, self-development. The ideal the Master recommended, and which was subsequently adopted as a standard, was expressed by the term "*jūn zí,*" which has been translated into English by various translators in diverse and interesting ways. "Gentleman" is perhaps the most common, if not the most accurate. According to Confucius, the *jūn zí* (or "superior man" as translated by Baynes from Wilhelm's German version of the *Yì Jīng*), possessed a number of esoteric qualities which he enumerated in the *Dà Xué* and developed more fully in *Zhōng Yōng*.

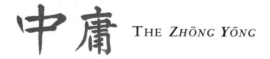 THE *ZHŌNG YŌNG*

When we talk of the root of Chinese culture and civilization, nothing comes closer to a verbal description than the phrase "*zhōng yōng*." What does this phrase mean? As we discussed in Chapter One, the Chinese developed a linguistic predilection for a concise, condensed precision of expression. There is perhaps no greater example of this than the phrase *zhōng yōng*. It contains a whole outlook and approach to living that is central to the Chinese way of thinking and the Chinese way of life.

WHO CAN RIDE THE DRAGON?

The modern character *zhōng* appears as 中. In essence, the character means "central," but through its uses and the various meanings that have derived, *zhōng* has taken on many profound connotations. Thus, as we have mentioned, China in the words of its native population is *zhōng guó*, the central country. In medicine, *zhōng*, the center, is the focus of the earth phase of five-phase theory.

Much of the deeper meaning of *zhōng* derives from its use in the phrase *zhōng yōng*. The significance of the word *zhōng* in this phrase modifies and amplifies its inherent meaning so that the character *zhōng* itself has the flavor of the phrase *zhōng yōng*. The meaning of *yōng* in this phrase acts to expand and emphasize the meaning of *zhōng*.

Taken alone, *yōng* means "normal," "not outstanding," "not particularly good, not particularly bad." The phrase *zhōng yōng* can be literally understood to mean "in the middle and not sticking out." It is a phrase which is commonly used to describe an approach to conduct that favors leaning neither to one side nor the other but staying in the center. Don't agree, don't disagree; *zhōng yōng*.

Another translation of the phrase could be, "Follow the middle way and don't attract attention." It is common to find Chinese children who have been taught this attitude by their fathers and mothers. "If you speak out, who knows what sort of trouble you might cause. Keep silent and you will harm no one." These words, according to one close Chinese friend, were the very ones used to instruct her in the discipline of correct conduct. They echo a phrase from the Confucian commentaries on the *Yì Jīng*, which resound in the passages of the *Zhōng Yōng*. In the text, Confucius speaks of the way of the superior man:

> The master man finds the center and does not waver; the mean man runs counter to the circulation about the invariable. The master man's axis does not wobble. The man of rare breed finds this center in season, the small man's center is rigid, he pays attention to the times and seasons, precisely because he is small and lacking all reverence. He said, "Center oneself in the invariable." Some have managed to do this, they have hit the true center, and then? Very few have been able to stay there.

This theme runs throughout the entire text, as seen in the following brief quotations:

> He stands firm in the middle of what whirls without leaning on anything either to one side or the other. The man of breed pivots himself on the unchanging and has faith.

The meaning of *zhōng yōng* is an amplification of the importance of centrality, the middle way. The character has an enlarged sense that incorporates this expanded idea. This sheds additional light on the significance of the Chinese name of their homeland: Zhōng Guó, the land of the middle way. To be Chinese is to pivot on this center.

Another major theme of the text is the process and devotion to the acquisition of knowledge and the attainment of a state of existence in which this knowledge is allowed to develop and take charge of one's affairs, of one's entire life. This devotion to knowledge and the processes whereby one comes into possession of it are centrally important to Confucianism and the role it has played throughout the development of Chinese civilization.

Indeed, the *Zhōng Yōng* opens with the following words:

> *What heaven has disposed and sealed is called the inborn nature. The realization of this nature is called the process. The clarification of this process [the understanding or making intelligible of this process] is called education.*

The influence of these Confucian ideas has proven to be deep and long lasting. In these words we find the germ of the entire system of education and examination for the civil servants who effectively ruled China for 2000 years. Taken together, these two essential concepts of the *Zhōng Yōng* can be paraphrased as follows: through study and learning, one can gain knowledge of conditions and discern the middle way; through holding steadfastly to this middle way and not seeking to exert extreme influence, one can conserve and cultivate one's knowledge and one's survival, thus contributing in the most effective way possible to the health and wellbeing of the whole country.

Many Western scholars who have studied Chinese civilization in its various aspects, perhaps most notably Joseph Needham, pose the question, "Why did China, possessed of great wisdom and technological prowess at such an early date, fail to develop modern science as in the West?" There are several answers to this questions, many of which cite the philosophical influence of the Confucians and particularly the neo-Confucians of the Song dynasty as likely candidates for the cause of this shortcoming. It seems to us, however, that such questioning misses the point. Indeed, it is like asking why a man setting out for New York fails to arrive in Chicago. He simply wasn't headed there.

WHO CAN RIDE THE DRAGON?

If our metaphor has merit, it is to effectively show that a class of Confucian scholars who administrated Chinese authority, charted and steered a course of gradual, restrained, and sustainable development for over 2000 years. The map for this course can be found in *Zhōng Yōng.* Its influence in Chinese thinking and Chinese life is virtually all-pervasive.

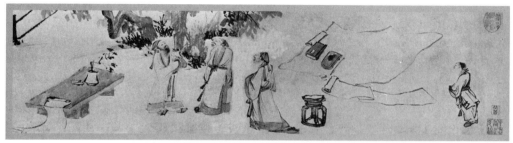

"The Noble Scholars," handscroll by T'ang Yin

Perhaps a more productive line of questioning is for Westerners to ask how Chinese civilization managed to survive the endless cycles of invasion, revolution, destruction and reconstruction that have characterized its millennial history. Certainly China has gone through periods of enormous hardship during which social values and standards have declined. At times in China's past, the suffering of her citizens has equaled or surpassed any in human history. Yet China survives. And it is this unparalleled survival that prompts us to ask not, "Why has China failed to become like Western nations?" but rather, "What has kept her moving steadily forward against tides of history that have crushed and washed away other ancient cultures?" Without a doubt, China's ancient culture survives today, changing as it has throughout its long history, but surviving nevertheless.

There is no better starting place to look for the answers to this question than in the *Zhōng Yōng* and the other literary classics we have discussed here. To understand the philosophical background of medical theories and healthcare strategies, we could do far worse than to study the *Zhōng Yōng.* Conversely, to understand China's long-term survival, we must comprehend the significant role traditional medicine has played in achieving that survival. Indeed, for a civilization to have endured as China has, it must have developed a workable system of caring for the health of its people. For if the people perish, there is no civilization or culture.

At the core of China's ancient native healthcare system is the concept of an orderly and harmonious arrangement of the people. This has always been understood to apply to people as individuals, people as entities in the natural environment, and people as social beings in the context of their civilization. The concept of balance in medical terms can be understood as an expression of an ideal which has been substantially shaped by the texts and interpretations of Confucian writers. The place of honor accorded to the *Zhōng Yōng* is evidence of the value and workability that Chinese scholars—including Chinese doctors—have discovered in its pages. These discoveries abide there, to be received by those who seek them.

CHAPTER FIVE

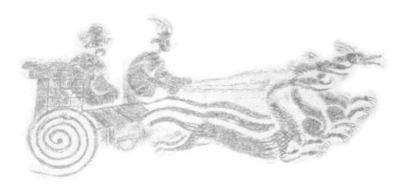

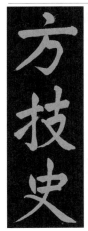

The Chinese Scientific Tradition

Scientific knowledge, like language, is intrinsically the common property of a group or else it is nothing at all. To understand it we need to know the special characteristics of the group that creates and applies it.

—THOMAS KUHN, *THE STRUCTURE OF SCIENTIFIC REVOLUTIONS*

Here we are brought up against the social and economic questions because they are exceedingly important for the comparative study of Chinese and Occidental science, technology, and medicine. It is probably impossible to understand the situation without realizing the enormous differences in social and economic structure between traditional China and the traditional West.

—JOSEPH NEEDHAM, LECTURE AT CHINESE UNIVERSITY OF HONG KONG, 1981

CHINA HAS PLAYED MANY ROLES in the drama of human history. Foremost among these is its age-old role as the birthplace of important scientific and technological developments. These have spread throughout the world over the many centuries of China's interactions with the West and other parts of the globe. From the Chinese, the West adopted such fundamental scientific and technological advancements as the compass, paper, printing, gunpowder, silk, porcelain, and binary mathematics, to name a few that illustrate the wide range of advances resulting from scientific study in China.

We will investigate the scientific traditions of China from several angles. First, an overview, drawing largely from the works of the great British sinologist Joseph Needham, whose massive, multivolume work, *Science and Civilization in China,* remains one of the most complete sources of information and understanding about science and civilization in China that Western academia has yet produced. In his introduction to a series of lectures given in 1981 in Hong Kong, Needham had the following to say on the subject of science in traditional China:

> *Before the river of Chinese science flowed, like all other such rivers, into the sea of modern science, China had seen remarkable achievements in many directions. For example, take mathematics: decimal place value and a blank space for the zero had begun in the land of the Yellow River earlier than anywhere else, and a decimal metrology had gone along with it. By the -1st century, Chinese artisans were checking their work with sliding calipers decimally graduated.*

Mathematics in ancient China occupied an important place in the intellectual community. The *Nine Chapters on the Mathematical Art (Jiŭ Zhāng Suàn Shù)* appeared in the Han Dynasty (206 B.C.E.–220 C.E.) summarizing the development of mathematics until that time. For two thousand years it has remained one of the oldest known and most respected books of mathematical problems and solutions in China.

Needham cited numerous other examples of the achievements of traditional sciences in China:

> *Three branches of physics were particularly well developed in ancient and mediaeval China: optics, acoustics, and magnetism. This was in striking contrast with the West, where mechanics and dynamics were relatively advanced but magnetic phenomena almost unknown.*

He also pointed out several notable differences between the development of scientific thought and artifacts in China and the West.

> *One most significant point is that although the Chinese of the Chou and Han, contemporary with the Greeks, probably did not rise to such heights as they, nevertheless in later centuries there was nothing at all in China corresponding to the Dark Ages in Europe. This fact is demonstrated well by the sciences of geography and cartography.*

WHO CAN RIDE THE DRAGON?

In addition to measuring and mapping the earth, ancient Chinese scientists focused their attention on the heavens and made observations and calculations of the motions of stars and planets. It is a curious fact that the Chinese approach to the study of the night sky permitted ancient astronomers in China to understand and chart the movements of planets and comets centuries before their counterparts in the West. In the early Han Dynasty a work appeared called *Zhōu Bì Suàn Jīng* that summarized this work and laid the foundation for the science of astronomy in China. It contains a theory of the heavens including a statement of the Pythagorean theorem for use in surveying and astronomy. This book contains the earliest known proof of this fundamental principle of mathematics.

Moving on to the area of applied sciences, Needham remarked:

> *Mechanical engineering, and indeed engineering in general, were fields in which classical Chinese culture scored special triumphs. Both forms of efficient harness for equine animals, a problem of link-work essentially, originated in the Chinese culture area. There, too, water power was first used for industry, about the same time as in the West, in the +1st or -1st century, not, however, for grinding cereals, but rather for the operation of metallurgical bellows. And that brings up something else, because the development of iron and steel technology in China constitutes a veritable epic, with the mastery of iron casting occurring some fifteen centuries before its achievement in Europe.*

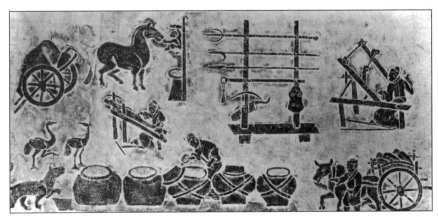

Rubbing from a Han Dynasty tomb in Peng Xian County, Sichuan Province which shows various technologies including winemaking, weaponry, butchery, weaving, and transportation

In martial technology the Chinese people also showed notable inventiveness. The first appearance of gunpowder occurred in China in the +9th century, and from +1000 onward there was a vigorous development of explosive weapons some three centuries before they were known in the West. Turning from the military to civilian, other aspects of technology have great importance, especially that of silk, in which the Chinese people excelled so early. Here the mastery of textile fibers of extremely long staple appears to have led to several fundamental engineering inventions, for example the first development in any civilization of the driving belt and the chain drive.

It is also possible to say that the first appearance of the standard method of inter-conversion of rotary and longitudinal motion, which found its great use in the early steam engines in Europe, came up also in connection with the metallurgical blowing-engines referred to already. If one were going in for epigrams, I ought to have mentioned when speaking of magnetism and of the magnetic compass that in China people were worrying about the nature of the declination (why the needle does not usually point exactly to the north) before Europeans had even heard about the polarity.

Nor was there any backwardness in the biological field either, because we find many agricultural inventions arising from an early time. I do not know how many of us are conscious of the fact that the first case of insects' being set to destroy other insects, and so work in the service of man, occurred in China: in the Nan Fang Ts'ao Mu Chuang written about +340, there is a description of how the farmers in Kuangtung and the southern provinces in general, who grow oranges in groves to convey to the marketplace at the right time of the year, purchase little bags containing a particular kind of ant, which they then hang on the orange trees. These ants completely keep down all the mites and spiders, and other insect pests, which would otherwise damage the orange crop.

On the subject of medicine, Needham had this to say in his lecture:

Medicine, again, is a field which it is rather absurd to bring up in a couple of minutes, because one could speak not for one hour, but many hours, on the subject of the history of medicine in China. It represents a field which aroused the intense interest of Chinese people all through the ages, and one which was developed by their special genius along lines perhaps more different from those of Europe than in any other case.

WHO CAN RIDE THE DRAGON?

In light of these remarks, it can be clearly seen that medicine in China developed in an atmosphere of intense scientific study, research, and development. It is important to recognize that, where the standards and customary practices of scientific investigation were distinctly different from those of modern science in the Western world, nevertheless such standards have existed in China for centuries. Thus ancient medical theorists and practitioners had the benefit of not only rich philosophical texts and other literary sources, but well established scientific theories and practices.

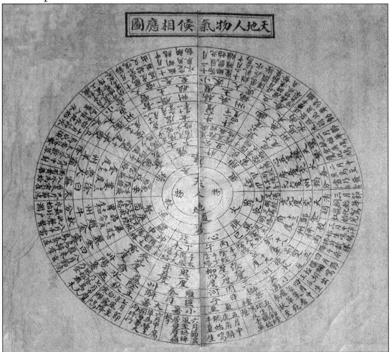

Chart from the Wings of the Classified Canon, depicting the relationship between the Yì Jīng and medicine, showing of the conditions of the systematic correspondence of the circulation of qì in humankind and material substances

As with each of the subjects treated in the foregoing sections of this book, the history of the scientific tradition in China is far too vast to permit comprehensive discussion here. The essential point is that medical theories arose from a complex matrix of intellectual investigation and scientific research in ancient China.

Beyond this, we will investigate two sources of medical traditions throughout Chinese history. These we have termed "Folk Medicine" and "Court Medicine." A more complete description of each follows.

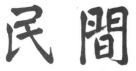 FOLK MEDICINE

In the summer of 1994, we traveled in the countryside of Western Sichuan province. Moving from village to village over the course of several weeks, we visited with friends, relatives of friends, friends of relatives, friends of friends.

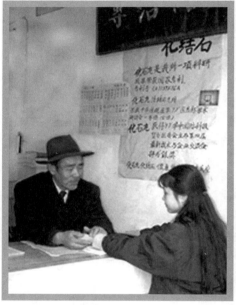

A local doctor palpates a patient's pulse

One stop we always made was at the local clinic. The logistics of providing healthcare for 1.2 billion people loom as one of the greatest challenges facing the leadership of the People's Republic of China today. In fact, enormous strides in the direction of providing safe, affordable, and effective healthcare to the masses of Chinese people have been made in recent decades. In the cities, more and more modern hospitals are appearing. But in the countryside, much of what exists in the way of medical facilities is pitifully primitive judged against Western standards. In places, it is not much different today than it has been for many centuries.

Yet today, even in the humblest surrounds, doctors hold forth against the constant onslaught of disease and injury using methods that their ancestors developed thousands of years ago alongside any and all the modern medical techniques and substances they can acquire. Our frequent visits to these clinics left an indelible impression of the spirit of medicine in the Chinese countryside. The following description of a clinic in Na Mu township located in Peng Xian County, just west of Chengdu, is typical.

An open door admits to a room approximately one-and-a-half by two-and-a-half meters. Behind a rickety writing desk sits an old man. His head is tilted at an angle, supported by his left hand. His eyes are

WHO CAN RIDE THE DRAGON?

only half open. He seems to be staring into some internal space. The first three fingers of his right hand are gently pressed against the radial artery on the wrist of a young woman who sits opposite him. She has a worried look on her face, which markedly contrasts the doctor's calm facade.

It is hot during the summer in Sichuan; hot and damp. Temperatures frequently push into the high thirties and low forties (Celsius) and the humidity must exceed 100 percent. The air drips with heat. In addition to the doctor and his patient, the tiny room is packed with several other villagers patiently waiting to see the doctor, and now us. We stand silently watching the diagnosis proceed. When the doctor raises his head from his contemplative pose and notices us, there is a momentary bustling. We manage at last to convince him it is not necessary to get us either chairs or tea and encourage him to simply return to his work. We have all day. We can talk and visit when he's done.

He proceeds in his examination, now noticeably more animated. The woman is suffering from an invasion of dampness and heat in the lower *jiào*. This, he points out to us, is analogous to the Western diagnosis of bacterial infection in the large intestines. He takes a pad of gossamer paper and writes out a prescription for a formula of Chinese herbs. To emphasize the importance of one particular ingredient he explains that it only grows in the local area. He collects it himself from the river banks. He offers to take us to a place where it grows abundantly to show it to us in its natural habitat and to pick some for us if we would like to have it.

"It is a very important herb," he repeats several times. "Very valuable."

The next patient takes his place in front of the old man. We learn later that the doctor is 77 years old. But his medical skills are "very poor," he confesses, compared to his father and especially his great-great grandfather. "He was one of those who could heal patients without leaving his study," he says in hushed, reverential tones. He points at us intensely with one finger: "*Qì*," he says by way of explaining how this could be accomplished. "He could transmit his *qì*."

He proceeds to examine the young peasant who now sits before him in obvious pain. The radius of his left arm has been broken by a load of bricks that fell from his cart while he was loading it, just a few hours earlier.

"No x-ray," smiles the old doctor. "Just treatment."

He takes the young man to the back of the clinic through a little connecting doorway. He holds aside the muslin drape that hangs across the doorway to invite us along to watch the treatment.

He calls out the names of several Chinese herbs and a young woman who had been drowsing with her head down on a table in the back of the house sleepily begins to mix up the formula, carefully tapping powder from several small glass vials into a porcelain cup. The old doctor then carefully palpates the young man's broken arm. It is only after several minutes of this examination that we realize the patient, who must be in excruciating pain, is evidencing none of it. Aside from an occasional wince and quiet one-word responses to the doctor's sporadic questions, the young man sits in silence as the examination proceeds.

"A dislocating fracture," says the doctor a few moments later. "No problem."

The assistant, probably a grandchild, arrives with the porcelain cup, which is now filled with a redolent blend of herbs, honey, and wine. It steams for a few moments while the doctor lets it cool. He takes the opportunity to address us directly.

"No problem," he says, "watch."

With one smooth movement he sets the broken bone, palpating the arm one last time to check his work. Satisfied, he proceeds with the treatment. Taking the preparation of herbs and honey, he mixes in more wine to get the consistency he wants. Then he makes a poultice and applies it to the young man's forearm. He uses two stiff pieces of an old cardboard box as a splint and fastens them together with shreds of white cotton fabric. Then he takes a larger piece of fabric and folds it into a triangle with which he binds up the patient's arm in a sling. The whole procedure takes just a few minutes. The grateful and, incredibly, smiling patient leaves the room.

We spent many afternoons in such settings, asking questions, observing, now and then providing treatment under the direction of such doctors to a steady stream of patients in clinic after clinic. In the clinic described above, the fee for a visit with the doctor was fifty Chinese cents, the equivalent of approximately six cents in American currency. Medicines, of course, are additional. A week's prescription for the woman with "damp heat in the lower *jiāo*" would cost her less than the equivalent of two US dollars, including the costly local specialty.

WHO CAN RIDE THE DRAGON?

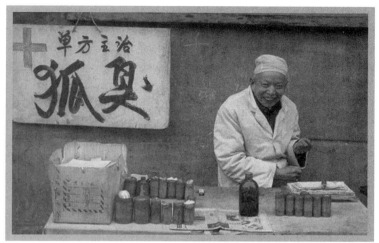
*An old country doctor at a roadside stand offers to treat offensive
body odors with a variety of herbal formulas*

In experiences like these we see images of the way medicine has
been practiced in the Chinese countryside for generations upon countless generations. Families of medical practitioners have continued for
hundreds if not thousands of years. One of the great credentials and
great boasts of a doctor of traditional Chinese medicine is that he or she
comes from a long line of medical experts. Such pedigrees are often
hard to document. Yet there can be little doubt of the fact that for thousands of years, medicine has been handed down from father to son,
from master to apprentice, in villages throughout the vast Chinese
countryside.

Thus it is an enormously complex task to describe Chinese "traditional medicine" in terms of its varieties and their origins. The problems related to comprehending the meanings of such a complex history are made even more difficult by several facts. For one, these family
traditions are often jealously guarded secrets. For another, it can be
difficult to distinguish between valid (i.e., effective) medical proce-
dures and substances, and pure hoax—just as in any place, at any
time, there is unfortunately an abundance of the latter compared to a
relative scarcity of the former. Moreover, it is undoubtedly true that
amongst the multiplicity of indigenous medical traditions China has
witnessed in its long history, there are as yet undiscovered medical
treasures to be found, understood, developed, and made accessible to
patients around the world.

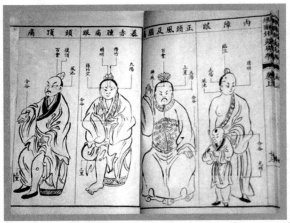

Illustration from Study of Acupuncture, Moxibustion and Yì Jīng (from left): "Blindness due to internal obstruction"; "Central head wind and headache"; "Extremely red and swollen eyes"; "Headache on the top of the head"

Towards such an end we suggest that an appreciation of the nature and characteristics of this "folk medicine" is an important step. Inevitably, the movement of people and ideas which has occurred throughout Chinese history has naturally blurred the distinction between traditions of healing that flourished in the countryside and those that developed under Imperial mandate.

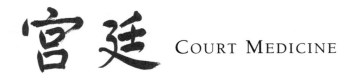 COURT MEDICINE

The distinction we make between "folk medicine" and "court medicine" does not necessarily imply differences in quality or authenticity of either. Rather, we wish to point out that while traditional theories and practices have continued evolving and developing in the countryside over thousands of years, there has also been a well-organized development of the subject conducted by successive official administrations. It is this latter tradition that we have termed "court medicine" simply to identify it as the result of efforts undertaken within the Imperial court under the aegis of Imperial authority.

There are several reasons for making this distinction, the primary one being to recognize the fundamental influence that any "official" compilation of a subject can exert. By the very nature of such compilation, the subject is edited and configured in ways that conform to the various needs, wants, and predilections of the authority that empowers those performing the work. As with many of the numerous other influences we have cataloged and discussed in this book, these influences range from minutely subtle to overwhelming in importance. In

WHO CAN RIDE THE DRAGON?

this section we present a general picture of the official or court tradition of Chinese medicine as it developed from one period to the next.

The officially canonized version of Chinese medicine can be seen to begin with the compilation of the *Yellow Emperor's Canon of Internal Medicine*. Its oldest extant versions date to the -2nd century B.C.E. In both form and content this work established the paradigm for officially recognized theories and practices of medicine in China. Though there are older medical texts—for example, the *Book of Rites* which includes records of Imperial medicine and clinical practices—the *Yellow Emperor's Canon* became the standard and the model for the field. (See Chapter 4 for a more complete discussion of this book.)

In the year 5 C.E. during the Han Dynasty, the court issued an official order for all scholars in the field of medicinal herbs to assemble from throughout the entire country. Then in 31 C.E. the Emperor Han Cheng Di issued an Imperial edict establishing the position of the court's official herbalist, the *Běn Cǎo Dài Zhāo*.

Though there were other major developments of court medicine over the next several hundred years, for now we skip forward in time to the Tang Dynasty. In 657 C.E. the Tang government ordered Shu Jin, who was then the chief official scholar, to confer with his colleagues and compose the first official pharmacopoeia, the *Táng Běn Cǎo*. This book not only established the beginning of what became a long tradition of such officially sanctioned compilations of medicinal substances in China, it exerted a tremendous influence in other countries as well, finding its way to Japan and Korea where it was taken as the standard on the subject of herbal ingredients.

Several decades earlier, in 624 C.E., the Tang throne had established the Tài Yī Shǔ to serve as the educational center for the study of medicine. Based on the educational structure of the Sui Dynasty (581–618 C.E.), it developed into a high-quality medical education center. It thus became one of the earliest schools of medicine in human history. Such achievements reflected the overall atmosphere of scientific advancement that was prevalent during the Tang period. The science of medicine had unique status among the various sciences that were fostered by Imperial authority.

In the period of the Northern Song, the government strengthened and improved the system of public health administration. Medical education was differentiated from healthcare delivery for administrative purposes. The Song government established the Hàn Lín Yī Guān Yuàn as the agency responsible for the administration of public health and the Tài Yī Jú as the agency empowered to control medical education. As part of this refinement of medical administration, the government also established a standardized examination required of all officially entitled doctors.

The Song court was also the origin of the Yào Jú, which was the official administrative agency for the management of herbal medicine. With this pattern of increasing specialization in terms of administrative responsibilities, the various sub-specialties of traditional medicine flourished in the Song as never before. The development and widespread use of ready-prepared medicines (*zhōng chéng yào*) increased rapidly during this period.

At the root of this characteristic pattern of the Song court's approach to medicine was the establishment of the Tài Yī Jú, mentioned above, as a sub-structure of the Guó Zǐ Jiān, the national educational administration. Those who worked for the Tài Yī Jú could concentrate their efforts solely on medical education. This concentration brought about a rapid and unprecedented development of medicine.

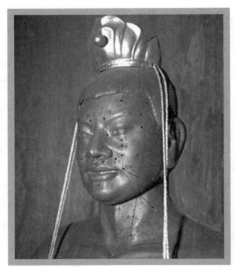

A copy of the bronze statue model, from the collection of Chengdu University of T.C.M.

In 1057, the Song government established the Jiào Zhèng Yī Shū Jú or Bureau of Rectifying Medical Texts to compile, correct, and reorganize the entire corpus of medical literature from throughout history, demonstrating their continued concentration on the development and refinement of medical science. It was also during the Song period that Wang Wei Yi built the now famous bronze model of the human body to clearly illustrate the location of the channels and network vessels and the points used for acupuncture and moxibustion.

This model has retained more than merely symbolic importance ever since. In the Ming Dynasty it was rebuilt and described in the *Tóng Rén Shū Xué Zhēn Jiǔ Tú Jīng (The Book of Illustrations of Acupuncture and Moxibustion Points of the Bronze Model)*. The Ming government also

WHO CAN RIDE THE DRAGON?

commissioned the writing of the *Yǒng Lè Dà Diǎn (Yong Le Encyclopedia),* an important reference book that gathered up essential material from numerous earlier works.

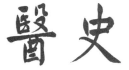

OVERVIEW OF THE HISTORICAL DEVELOPMENT OF MEDICINE IN CHINA

The main question that any doctor or patient asks about any form of medicine is, "Does it work?" In order to arrive at a positive answer to this question, it is useful to understand how Chinese medicine has developed throughout its long history. A brief timeline that begins more than 3000 years ago helps provide a sense of the dynamic historical development of traditional medicine in China. Medical historians in China typically break down this timeline into seven main periods. We have kept to this model as it reflects a more or less "organic" sense of the growth of the subject.

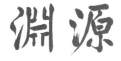

THE PERIOD OF ORIGINS (? −2100 B.C.E.)

This is the period of prehistory in China. Evidence to support conjectures and theories is scant. Yet it is possible to assemble images of humanity's struggle to survive in the face of overwhelming natural forces. This period witnessed the development of stone and bone implements, which may or may not have included precursors of acupuncture needles. It was also the period in which agriculture appeared, providing the basis for stable cultural development. Discovery of the properties and functions of various herbs, minerals, and animals played a role of primary importance with respect to the development of medicine.

It was during this prehistoric period that the three legendary Emperor-Gods of China were said to have existed. Fu Xi, Shen Nong, and Huang Di (the Yellow Emperor) each brought forth essential elements of culture in China that allowed the long saga of Chinese civilization to begin. Fu Xi invented the institution of marriage, setting man and woman into their natural relationship and stabilizing patterns of reproduction and group survival. As mentioned earlier, Fu Xi also established the signs of the *Yì Jīng*, the *bā guà* or eight trigrams, thus setting in place and into motion the fundamental principles of Chinese thought.

The next of these legendary kings of prehistoric China was Shen Nong. His role in the development of civilization is clearly recorded in his name, which means "God of Agriculture." It was Shen Nong who invented the pattern, as well as the earliest implements, of farming in China. According to legend, it was also Shen Nong who sampled hundreds of different plants, divining their tastes, properties, and medicinal functions, and setting herbal medicine on a path that it has followed ever since. The same principle of classifying herbal ingredients according to their taste, *qì*, and other essential properties and functions is used in modern herbal pharmacies and clinics.

But it was the not until the time of the Yellow Emperor, Huang Di, the third of these legendary figures, that Chinese civilization was fully synthesized and established in its proper course. Huang Di is regarded, therefore, as the first true Emperor of China.

It was in the name of the Yellow Emperor, moreover, that the subject and the study of medicine was first codified. As mentioned earlier in Chapter 4, the conversations between Huang Di and his chief physician, Qi Bo, form the corpus of a work, the *Yellow Emperor's Canon of Internal Medicine,* compiled and refined over a period of centuries, that has endured as the keystone of medical theory in China.

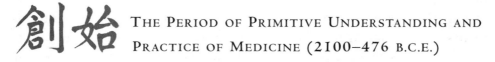 THE PERIOD OF PRIMITIVE UNDERSTANDING AND PRACTICE OF MEDICINE (2100–476 B.C.E.)

This period witnessed the growth and development of civilization, culture, philosophy, and science in China. It was during these 1500 years or so that the Chinese learned to understand their natural environment and particularize this understanding in large numbers of scientific and technological artifacts. There appeared instruments such as the *guī*, with which the period of the solstices could be established. It was also a period that witnessed the compilation of great literary classics such as the *Book of Songs* and the *Annals of the Spring and Autumn*. Lao Zi wrote the *Dào Dé Jīng* and left it with a gatekeeper at the pass that led beyond civilization back to the unalloyed natural world that he so earnestly sought.

WHO CAN RIDE THE DRAGON?

In the field of medicine, several important developments occurred. Magician doctors known as *wū* or shamans (see Chapter Two) appeared and rose to prominence in the Shang Period (1520–1039 B.C.E.). Evidence suggests that these powerful sorcerers and necromancers virtually ruled the land during much of this period. Standing as messengers between the world of mankind and the mysterious unseen realm of the gods, the *wū* were able to wield enormous social and political power. The "emperors" were called the "sons of heaven," and since the *wū* stood between man and heaven, they occupied a position of pivotal importance in each and every kingdom that rose and fell during this period.

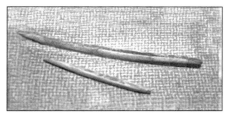

Ancient bone needles, from the collection of the Chengdu University of T.C.M.

One primary way this power was made manifest was in the healing rituals the *wū* performed. As noted earlier, many of the fundamental notions about the origin and treatment of disease stem from this period. Powerful unseen forces—spirits, demons, and the like—were understood as the causes of disease. It was the work of the *wū* to rid the afflicted by way of magical intervention. These interventions took the form of word magic, dance rituals, herbal concoctions, and a whole array of other primitive techniques. Indeed, it was a time of primitive powers, which gave way to the beginnings of the Feudal Age with the establishment of the Zhou Dynasty.

During the Zhou period (1066–770 B.C.E.) the seeds of humanistic philosophy began to grow. The principle of the Zhou rulers was contained in the phrase, "respect heaven but protect the people." One Zhou ruler is reported to have said, "Heaven cannot be trusted. Heaven must conform to the will of the people." Such a change in attitude gave rise to the organized search for the origins and principles of natural phenomena. It was during this time and particularly in the period known as Spring and Autumn, that the fundamental theories of Chinese indigenous naturalistic philosophy began to bloom. This concern for the well-being of the people manifested in an intensification of efforts to study and develop medical theories and techniques.

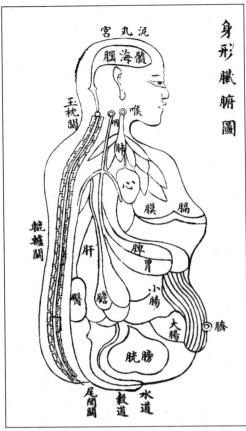

身形臟腑圖

宮丸泥
腦海髓
玉枕關
喉
䐃
肺
心
轆轤關
膜 膈
肝
脾胃
腎 膽
小腸
大腸
臍
胱膀
尾閭關 穀道 水道

A Qing Dynasty rendition of the principal internal organs, showing a physiological schema adopted more than 2000 years ago

The theories of yīn and yáng, the five phases, and *qì*—the fundamental components of the theoretical infrastructure of Chinese medicine—were developed and synthesized. The concepts of *jīng, qì, shén, xuè* (essence, *qì*, spirit, and blood) also appeared, as did the notion of the five viscera and six bowels.

Thus we can see that some 2500 years ago, the basic framework of medical theory—the two paradigms that form the basis of all theories of Chinese internal medicine—appeared and began to develop in China.

Also during this period the techniques of decocting medicinal herbs came into widespread use. This was an important step in the development of herbal science, as it was the ability to formulate complex prescriptions that allowed early pharmacists to explore and develop the synergistic properties of herbal ingredients which form the essence of the science of formula writing, preparation, and utilization—all practiced to this day.

By the end of the Spring and Autumn period, there were collections of herbal ingredients that ran into the hundreds, although there was apparently no comprehensive text of herbal science. However, public health organizations, and the concept of specialization in medicine, were innovations that did emerge. A system was organized that installed a Chief Physician whose position was roughly analogous to the contemporary Director of Public Health. This doctor directed the activities of all other officially recognized practitioners, dividing them according to three levels of accomplishment and skill. In this organization, there was a separate department of herbal medicine, a department of medical equipment, and, inevitably, an accounting department.

This same organizational system also gave rise to the first department of nursing. It included, among its various documentary requirements, the issuance of death certificates. Doctors in this system were required to pass annual reviews, not only of their knowledge and skill but also of their accomplishments during the previous year. A doctor's salary level was set according to the results of this yearly review. Many of the advances of medicine during the successive period, and in the Qin Dynasty particularly, are a result of the value placed in this administrative system.

原理 CODIFICATION OF THE BASIC THEORIES AND SYSTEMS OF MEDICINE (475 B.C.E–265 C.E.)

This is the period commonly referred to as the Early Stage of the Feudal Age of Chinese history. It is however important to note that the meaning of feudalism in China is characteristically different than what is commonly understood as feudalism in the traditions of the West. Again, we quote from Joseph Needham:

> *It is probably impossible to understand the situation without realizing the enormous differences in social and economic structure between traditional China and the traditional West. Although many differences of interpretation exist among scholars, I feel quite satisfied with the broad principle that during approximately the past two thousand years, China did not have feudalism in the aristocratic military Western sense. ... It was certainly something different from what Europe knew.*

In 221 B.C.E. the first emperor of Imperial China established a unified, multinational state under a centralized leadership for the first time in Chinese history. His reign witnessed the achievement of standards in many fields, including law, economic and financial exchange, written language, and weights and measures. These societal standardizations led to previously unattainable levels of stability. Thus a period of several hundred years of productive and prosperous times ensued, built upon a background of Imperial policy that fostered production in both agriculture and manufacturing.

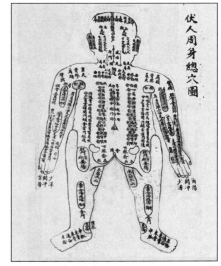

Ancient chart showing a posterior view of the acupuncture points on the body

With the previously unknown levels of social and economic achievements there came a commensurate increase in the demand for cultural and philosophical organization and artifacts. In all fields—science and learning, philosophy and politics—there were high levels of achievement. Such developments had a profound and lasting influence on the development of medicine in China.

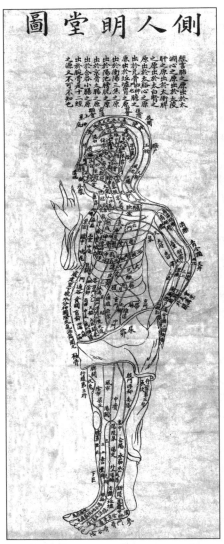

Chart of acupoints that accompanies a discussion of the circulation of *qì* through the channels and network vessels

First and foremost, this resulted in a codification of philosophical and medical theories such as yīn-yáng theory and the theory of the five phases. Of special importance was the thorough synthesis of the theories of *jīng, qì, and shén*. This synthesis, along with methods of preserving health, maintaining youth, and lengthening life, was later transplanted into the field of medicine from Daoism. With this blending of theory there came a long-lasting association between the Daoist alchemists and chemists and the medical specialists. The Daoist principles of cultivation of *jīng* and *qì* to nourish *shén* became enshrined within the corpus of traditional Chinese medical theory. The Daoist search for the internal elixir became the concern of medical specialists as well.

The greatest artifact of this period of codification of medical theory is the *Huáng Dì Nèi Jīng (Yellow Emperor's Canon of Internal Medicine)*. As described in Chapter 4, this work set forth the blueprint of the infrastructure of Chinese medical theories and methods. It is at the same time a profoundly philosophical text which reveals the concern of medical specialists of this period for the spiritual aspects of health and disease. Virtually all medical texts that have survived since this period owe much to the *Huáng Dì Nèi Jīng*; in fact, it is not an overstatement to say that they are based upon it.

WHO CAN RIDE THE DRAGON?

Herbology in particular flourished during the Han Dynasty. The Han Emperor Cheng established a civil service position of Herbalist, thereby providing the practical basis for the development of the study and profession of herbal pharmacy. At the same time, cultural exchange with India and Middle Eastern regions flourished along the Silk Road, bringing vast new bodies of herbal lore and knowledge to China. Foreign herbs were imported and included in the compilations of effective ingredients. This growth in herbal science resulted in the appearance of the first comprehensive text on the subject, entitled *Shén Nóng Běn Cǎo Jīng (Shen Nong's Classic of Herbology)*.

Another major contribution to the systematic development of Chinese medicine was the work of the famous Han Dynasty physician, Zhang Zhong Jing (see Chapter 4). His monumental work, the *Shāng Hán Lùn (On Cold Damage)* remains to this day the principal source for herbal prescriptions. This book presented the first systematic organization of the clinical practice of medicine. It set forth the principles of differential diagnosis. It laid the groundwork and achieved several important milestones in the study and treatment of febrile diseases. In China's modern universities of traditional medicine, there are departments dedicated solely to the study of this single book.

In the third century, the *Mài Jīng (Classic of the Pulse)* was written by Wang Shu He, an eminent doctor of the Han court. This book systematized the study of the pulse. It established the theory of the three primary positions for pulse-taking, laid out the principles of pulse diagnosis, and related these diagnostic principles to treatment protocols. To this day, the theory and practice of pulse diagnosis owes its essential characteristics to the contents of this book.

The literary root of the subject of acupuncture appeared at the end of the Warring States Period. This book, *Zhēn Jiū Jiǎ Yǐ Jīng (Acupuncture Celestial Root)* provided the basis for the development of acupuncture over the next thousand years. This book canonized the location of 647 acupuncture points. It also explained the basic theories and techniques of acupuncture. Its influence was felt outside China, as the book was exported to Japan, Korea, and other Asian countries where it served as the standard text on the subject.

Finally, it would not be possible to describe this period in the development of Chinese medicine without mentioning the famous Han Dynasty physician Hua Tuo, known in China as the father of external medicine. He established the basic principles and techniques of surgery and systematized treatment protocols for many external syndromes and ailments. His study of acupuncture anatomy resulted in the discovery of a special series of points along the upper spine which bear his name.

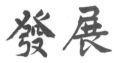 THE FULL DEVELOPMENT OF CHINESE MEDICINE: 265–960 C.E.

Let us recall the Chinese saying cited earlier: "Sometimes we're together; sometimes we're apart." It refers to, among other things, the pattern of unification and partition of the various states, dynasties, and regions of the country. During this period of time, the Three Kingdoms era at its beginning and the Five Dynasties period at its end, China was indeed both united and divided. There were roughly twenty different governments that ruled parts or all of the country at successive and overlapping times. Thus much of this period was characterized by relative instability, with the very notable exception of the Tang Dynasty.

The Tang rulers cultivated stability and prosperity, and in this period Chinese civilization rose to new heights, becoming the cultural center of Asia. Under the influence of this prosperity, the Chinese population flourished. Science and learning kept pace with social and economic developments. Chinese culture blossomed. This was reflected in the establishment of what may well be the world's oldest research center, Hán Lín Yuàn, built more than 1000 years before any such structure was to appear in Europe.

As noted in the overview given in Chapter 4, the three major religious traditions flourished as well. Confucianism, Daoism, and Buddhism were all popular; and their influence on the development of medicine increased. So, too, did the influence of Daoist chemists and alchemists, the most notable of whom, Sun Si Miao, made unequaled contributions to the sciences of chemistry and medicine. The contributions of the Buddhists to the development of medicine are not to be overlooked, for they brought the ancient traditions of Indian medicine and, importantly, herbal ingredients to the growing knowledge base of Chinese medicine. But it was the Confucians who exerted comprehensive influence over the development of medicine, as over Chinese social structures in general.

Since the days of the Han Dynasty, the Confucian school provided the ideological root for Chinese education and the civil service examination by means of which the mandarinate that administered the country was maintained. Foremost among the characteristics of this Confucian root were the concepts of humanity and justice. These two broad concepts were incorporated into the training of doctors and served as the basis for the moral cultivation of medical personnel. There originated what has become an old saying, "Medicine is the art of benevolence."

The developments that took place under these various influences resulted in an extension of medical knowledge, techniques, and, importantly, medical ethics that went far beyond the limits of earlier periods. It was a time of vast cultural and economic prosperity, and medicine developed to serve the people.

In the area of basic medical theory, the *Yellow Emperor's Canon of Internal Medicine* was rearranged by a number of eminent physicians of the Tang period into the form in which it is now known. They elaborated and explained the ancient passages, and in 610, there appeared for the first time a comprehensive curriculum for the study of the causes and symptoms of disease based upon this text.

Clinical medicine also experienced enormous developments. Foremost among these was the emergence of medical specializations. Departments of surgery, traumatology, pediatrics, and gynecology appeared as well as the earliest books on various specializations in medicine.

Perhaps the greatest advancement in the field of medicine, however, came in the field of herbal pharmacy. In 659, the Tang court conducted what amounted to a nationwide mobilization of resources in order to produce what may well be the world's oldest comprehensive pharmacopoeia, *Táng Běn Cǎo*. also known as the *Xīn Xiū Běn Cǎo*. To complete this book, research was conducted throughout China. Summaries of all available older books were produced and gathered together. The result was a comprehensive text of herbal medicine, which served not just Chinese but Japanese, Korean, Vietnamese, and other Asian nations' doctors, as well as becoming the standard, mandatory text on the subject. Indeed, there appeared at this time a number of such comprehensive texts on medicine, including a compendium of clinical medicine which contains the first references to smallpox and other communicable diseases such as tuberculosis.

As mentioned above, it was in this period that the great physician Sun Si Miao lived and worked. His book, *Qiān Jīn Fāng* (*Prescriptions Worth a Thousand Pieces of Gold*) is a digest of the medical knowledge of the time. He was a widely learned man who respected and studied all the major traditions of learning and philosophy available to him. In his book he gave particular attention to the special functional characteristics of herbs, stressing the importance of the geographical regions where herbs are grown in determining their medical effectiveness. He emphasized the importance of gynecology and more generally the cultivation and preservation of health and wellbeing. Even today, his book is widely respected and used as a guidebook for the practice of clinical medicine.

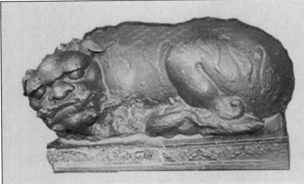

Immortal herb dog of Sun Si Miao

Sun Si Miao took his dog with him on countless expeditions to the mountains to gather medicinal herbs. Before tasting any sample collected, Sun Si Miao always broke off a bit and fed it to the dog. In time, the dog became so strong and healthy that it achieved immortality. Through the 19th century, tradditional pharmacists memorialized this story with statues of Sun Si Miao and his dog on their counters.

In approximately the fifth century C.E. the establishment of medical education appeared in China. By the seventh century, the Tang government created the Tài Yī Shǔ, the official government office of medicine. In this office, there existed a department devoted to medical education, which was further subdivided into four main areas of medical specialization: the department of medicine; the department of acupuncture; the department of massage and traumatology; and the department of incantation. This last department is evidence that the ancient roots of shamanistic medicine retained significant importance at this time.

The lengths of courses of study in various medical specializations were established: internal medicine required seven years; pediatrics, five years; external medicine, four years. With such standardization of the form and content of medical education and administration, the foundation was laid for a new era of development. However, the dictates and delimitations of governmental standardization primarily shaped Court Medicine. As the facilities of this official medical establishment in the Imperial Court were necessarily limited, the preponderance of medical training throughout this era remained in the purview of Folk Medicine, and held the form of the traditional master-apprentice relationship, beyond official control.

成就 OUTSTANDING ACHIEVEMENTS— BLAZING NEW TRAILS: 960–1368 C.E.

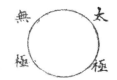
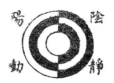
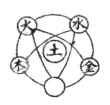
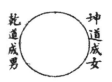

One of the defining aspects of this period was the constant warfare between the Han Chinese and the Mongols. The instability created by this continuous warfare ended in 1279 C.E. with the establishment of the Yuan (Mongol) Dynasty (1206–1368).

At the beginning of the Song Dynasty, however, there was a brief period marked by stability and economic development. As a result, science, particularly medical science, flourished. This period also saw the technological development and implementation of three of the most significant scientific advancements of the ancient world: gunpowder, the compass, and printing. The proliferation of printed materials in particular fostered the rapid growth and development of medical science in China and eventually throughout the whole world.

Many ancient medical compilations were edited and widely published. The Song government established an official printing house to oversee and produce corrected medical texts. This resulted in standard editions of such fundamentally important texts as the *Yellow Emperor's Canon of Internal Medicine,* the *Classic of Difficult Issues, Treatise on Cold Damage, Prescriptions from the Golden Cabinet,* the *Classic of Acupuncture and Moxibustion,* and *Prescriptions Worth a Thousand Pieces of Gold,* all mentioned in the foregoing sections.

In the field of ideology, the neo-Confucian movement developed enormous momentum and infused all schools of thought with a naturalistic rationalism that served as the basis for scientific thinking. In the field of medical theory, this influence was typified by the development of the theory of the five movements and the six influences. The term "five movements" referred to the cyclic interrelationships between the five phases. The "six influences" were understood to be six aspects of environmental causes of disease, namely wind, heat, damp, cold, dryness, and fire

Tài jí diagram from Xìng Mìng Guī Zhī:
1. *Tài jí comes from wú jí*
2. *Yīn stillness and yáng motion*
3. *The five phases*
4. *The way of kūn guà creates woman on the right side; the way of qián guà creates man on the left side*
5. *Everything on earth transforms and is born*

(summerheat). These concepts appeared in the ancient texts, especially the *Yellow Emperor's Canon,* but in the Song period they underwent an elaborate transformation to become the basis of a comprehensive and systematic theory of the causes and treatments of disease.

These concepts were blended together with other fundamental theoretical structures such as the Heavenly Stems and Earthly Branches (an ancient system of reckoning time according to an elaborate pattern of divisions of the lunar calendar) as well as the principles of astronomy and astrology, meteorology, and geography. Taken together, this comprehensive knowledge base served to provide explanations as well as predictions concerning causes and treatments for various diseases. The Song government annually published a "calendar of movements" based on this system which announced in advance what influences would be at play, what kinds of diseases could be expected to appear, and what sort of medicines and treatments should be administered.

This sort of publication, perhaps roughly analogous to our *Old Farmer's Almanac,* reflected the sophisticated levels of scholarship and debate in the field of medical studies. In this intellectual environment there emerged a number of thinkers who challenged ancient ideas, offering revisions to theories that had been accepted for centuries. Foremost among these was Wang An Shi, who lived during the Northern Song period. Succinctly stated, his philosophy was a harbinger of the "God is dead" school of thought. He held that there was no supreme God nor spirits or other "supernatural" forces. He purveyed the primacy of the natural law of yīn and yáng and the five phases.

The Song government continued to pursue a policy of separating public health administration and education. The chief administrative body was known as the Hàn Lín Yī Guān Yuàn; the institution of academic education in medicine was called Tài Yī Jú. These two separate structures helped refine the focus of medical study and application.

The Song government also made strides in the process of qualifications of medical specialists. A standardized exam, open to all who wished to apply, was conducted to determine the qualifications of individual practitioners. The development and application of strict standards greatly enhanced the level of medical knowledge and education. This drive for standards also resulted in the establishment of a branch of the medical administration devoted to the registration and quality control of herbal medicines, including patent formulas, marking the

WHO CAN RIDE THE DRAGON?

beginning of a tradition of Chinese prepared formulas (*zhōng chéng yào*) that continues to the present.

Compilation of the official pharmacopoeia flourished in this atmosphere. In the Tang Dynasty, the official compendium included some 850 medicinal substances. In the Song period, this more than doubled with the publication of an official listing of herbal ingredients numbering 1746.

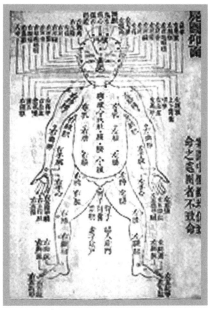

The Song Dynasty also witnessed the advent of a forensic medicine specialty. The principles of forensic medicine were already ancient, having first appeared in the third century C.E. with the introduction of medical evidence in trials at law. In the sixth century C.E., a book on the subject by Xue Zi Chai appeared. Unfortunately, this book has been lost. In 1247 C.E., Song Chi wrote what was to become the basic textbook on the subject, entitled *A Book to Wash Away Injustice*. It has been translated into many languages and has exerted enormous influence in the field.

Illustration from Xī Yuān Lùn (A Book to Wash Away Injustice), showing potentially fatal points

In general, the Song was a period of extraordinary growth and development in the sciences. Medical theorists, inspired by thinkers such as Wang An Shi, mentioned above, began to challenge ancient accepted beliefs. "Ancient formulas cannot treat all of today's diseases" became a rallying cry; and herbal pharmacy flourished as never before. Ironically, the advent of continuous warfare created an insatiable demand for effective medicines and medical treatments. This spurred the development of acupuncture as well as herbal pharmacy.

It was in this period that Wang Wei Yi devised the brass model of the human body which included both an internal section containing the five *zàng* and six *fǔ* organs, and an exterior section containing 657 acupuncture points. This standardized model greatly enhanced the quality of instruction and examination in acupuncture. It stimulated discussion and debate concerning the precise location, function, and effectiveness of the points.

With increased levels of scholarship and debate, there inevitably developed factions of medical thinking; and for the first time in Chinese medical history, distinct schools of thought appeared, each purveying differing sets of doctrines, different notions of the etiology of disease, and different strategies for treatment and preservation of health. Prior to the Tang and Song periods, such factionalization had not been prevalent. The work of Liu He Jian, however, served to foster the development of one of four contesting schools of thought.

Liu's theory was known as the "principle of heat." He held that all accumulations of *qì* would develop into heat and transform into fire. He regarded such pathogenic heat as the primary factor in the onset of disease in general but particularly injuries brought on by the cold. One clinical result of this theory was the preponderance of herbs that are cold in nature in formulas written by the Han Liang Pai, adherents of what came to be regarded as the Cold-ists school.

The second of these four schools, called the Xiāo Xià (Disperse Downwards) school, depended heavily on the work of Zhang Zi He. In treating disease in general, he advocated an approach to rid the body of pathogenic *qì*. This school formulated practices primarily focused on releasing the lower *jiāo*—generally, the organs of elimination. (See Chapter 7 for a definition of lower *jiāo*).

Li Dong Yuan authored a theory that emphasized the earth phase (one of the five phases) as the primary focus for medical intervention. Reasoning that everything developed from the element of the earth, this school of thought, known as the Bŭ Tŭ (Nourish the Earth) school, favored supplementation of the middle *jiāo* (the spleen and stomach or the digestive system).

Finally, Zhu Dan Xi became identified with a school of thought that heavily emphasized the importance of yīn as the nutritive, substantial aspect of the body on which all other functions depend. This school of thought, known as the Nourish the Yīn School, relied heavily on herbs that supplement and nourish the yīn.

Each of these four schools of thought evolved, engendering diverse approaches to clinical medicine. Perhaps most importantly, the atmosphere of contending scholars served to stimulate interest and activity in medical education, theory, and practice.

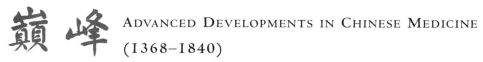

巅 峰 ADVANCED DEVELOPMENTS IN CHINESE MEDICINE (1368–1840)

This period of time saw the decline of Chinese feudalism and, eventually, the onset of the demise of the dynastic era of Chinese history. This end was not without its new beginnings. In fact, the period of the Ming and Qing dynasties saw numerous developments of Chinese civilization that were unequaled in earlier times.

Among the most impressive of such accomplishments were the voyages of Zheng He who, at the order of the Ming emperor, Cheng Zu, sailed to more than thirty countries, establishing political and economic relationships throughout the South China Sea and the Indian Ocean. A half-century or more before Columbus' famous voyage of discovery, Zheng He had accomplished a virtually unprecedented navigational feat.

One result of this high level of economic and political exchange was the influx of foreign cultural influences as well as foreign capital. But as China prospered in this period, the seeds of decay spread throughout the society.

This pattern of economic growth and development, accompanied by widespread social decay, continued with the establishment of the last dynasty, the Qing. The factors that brought about the ultimate downfall of more than 2000 years of dynastic tradition in China are complex and a proper treatment of them would lead us far beyond the scope of this book. In brief, corrupt and incompetent government over several generations resulted in an Imperial system that was overripe and beginning to rot. When the Opium Wars broke out in 1840, a step-by-step process was initiated that ended with the dissolution not only of the Qing court but also of the entire dynastic tradition.

Nonetheless, during the periods of stability that frequently occurred in the Ming and Qing eras, enormous advances in all fields of learning took place. In medicine, some particularly impressive steps were taken. Among these was the publication of the most comprehensive text of herbal pharmacy in history, the *Běn Cǎo Gāng Mù* by Li Shi Zhen. This book consisted of fifty-two volumes listing nearly two thousand kinds of herbs and over eleven thousand formulas. It contains more than a thousand illustrations and has a total of nearly two million words.

More important than its size was the fact that it focused extensively on pharmacological research, marking a turning point in the development of the materia medica. The author drew heavily on ancient sources in a wide variety of disciplines including botany, zoology, mineralogy, physiology, astrology, and meteorology. It was published in 1596 C.E. and soon circulated beyond China's borders into Japan, Korea, and other Asian countries.

Publication of medical books in this period took place at a rate exceeding that of any earlier period. Somewhat paradoxically, the policy prevalent throughout the Qing period was one of extremely conservative values, characterized by numerous efforts to control the work and even the thoughts of those engaged in such research and writing. The strictures of this conservative approach forced doctors to research carefully and develop systematically organized materials of medical treatment and pharmacology.

This led to many significant developments. As early as the middle of the sixteenth century, during the Ming Dynasty, vaccination methods first appeared. By the Qing Dynasty, use of these techniques had become common, requiring the establishment of an office within the public health structure to administer the official immunization programs.

Another breakthrough came in the 18th century with the publication of a book entitled *Correction in the Field of Medicine* (*Yī Lín Gǎi Cuò*) by Wang Qing Ren. Wang conducted extensive research on human anatomy, and his book corrected many previously held notions concerning gross anatomy. Correction and refinement were also on the minds of acupuncture specialists during this period, resulting in a number of texts that recodified the number and location of acupuncture points.

Of particular note is a book entitled *The Great Essence of Acupuncture and Moxibustion* (*Zhēn Jiǔ Jí Yīng*) by Gao Wu. In it he summarized the state of the art and science of acupuncture and moxibustion up through the 16th century. He also differentiated between men, women, and children regarding the location of points as well as treatment methods. He developed separate brass models of male, female, and children's bodies in order to standardize point locations.

The year 1522 saw the establishment of a standardized form for reporting on clinical case studies. A book entitled *Hán's General Survey on Medicine* (*Hán Shì Yī Tōng*) developed this standard form based upon

WHO CAN RIDE THE DRAGON?

historical models dating back to the Zhou period (1066–770 B.C.E.). This resulted in a move to standardize the format for clinical interviews as well as treatment protocols. In 1584, Wu Kun, in a book entitled *The Language of the Pulse (Mài Yǔ)*, laid down the following seven-method approach.

1. *Date, Location, Patient name;*

2. *Patient's age, body shape, color, sound;*

3. *What is the chief complaint and when did it begin?*

4. *What was the initial symptom? Was any medication given and to what effect?*

5. *At which time of day does the patient feel worse? Does the body prefer cold or heat? What are the pulses like?*

6. *Clearly establish the illness according to accepted texts: what is the root and what is the branch, that is, what needs to be treated first? What needs to be supplemented and what needs to be drained?*

7. *List the herbal formula itself, citing the classical formula plus any herbs added to or taken away from it, and clearly identifying the function of each primary ingredient.*

A Chinese medical association was formed in 1568 for the purpose of fostering exchange of ideas regarding classical texts, clinical experience, and other vital issues related to the education and practice of medicine. Known as the "House of the Human Community of Chinese Medicine," this affiliation of doctors provided its members with a forum for the development of their professional knowledge and skills.

At the end of the 18th century, the first medical journal appeared under the editorship of Tang Da Lie. This journal included articles covering a comprehensive range of theoretical and clinical topics and provided the medical community with still greater access to and exchange of ideas and methodologies.

In general, this period witnessed great advances in academic exchange between scholars and doctors. These exchanges extended far beyond China's borders, and Chinese medicine found its way not only into countries throughout Asia and the Middle East but into Europe as well.

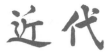

DEVELOPMENT OF CHINESE MEDICINE: 1840 TO THE PRESENT

After the middle of the 19th century, China entered a protracted period of economic, political, social, and cultural decline. As early as the seventeenth century, European missionaries, especially the Jesuits, brought knowledge of Western scientific developments. Within two centuries, Western medicine had begun to supplant traditional Chinese medicine in China. This period also marked the beginning of the integration of Western and Chinese medicine.

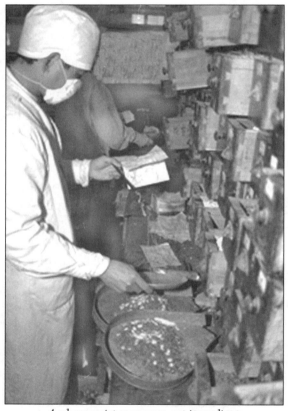

A pharmacist measures out ingredients for an herbal formula

However, as a result of fundamental disparities between these two medical approaches, as well as prevailing attitudes among Chinese intellectuals, various problems arose, and conflicting points of view developed as to their resolution. Briefly, some favored abandoning the ancient ways of traditional medicine and adopting the modern Western scientific methods. Others, typically those who were politically as well as culturally conservative, preferred to forego the benefits of modern medicine in favor of the orthodox traditional approach. A third faction (the pioneers of their day) proposed an integration of the two systems that would develop the strengths and buffer the weaknesses of each.

On the whole, Chinese medicine fared poorly throughout much of the closing decades of the 19th century and the opening decades of the 20th century. In 1925, the National Education Union tried to include Chinese medicine in the curricula of medical schools, but this effort was refused by the National government. Things grew bleaker still for traditional medicine when, in 1929, the National Committee on Public Health adopted a resolution to abolish Chinese medicine.

During the decade of their struggle to unify the country, the Communists in China championed traditional medicine for two main reasons. First, the Nationalists had taken a strong stance against traditional medicine. Second, traditional medicine offered the Communists the least expensive means for providing the most basic healthcare for large numbers of people. Thus, in the years following the success of the Communist revolution in 1949, traditional medicine in China began its modern resurgence. Mao Ze Dong himself spoke out on numerous occasions, exhorting his followers to develop the "great treasurehouse of Chinese medicine."

In the 1950's this policy was put into effect with the drafting of a corps of some 2000 medical doctors from around the country who were given the mandate to update, modernize, and develop traditional medicine. Four Colleges of Traditional Chinese Medicine were established, one in Beijing, one in Shanghai, one in Guangzhou, and one in Chengdu. These schools, as well as the dozens of other schools and colleges of T.C.M. that have come into being in more recent years, have undertaken the task of bringing this ancient form of medicine into the contemporary world. Now, as in ages past, it is a vast and complex job. Today, however, despite considerable adversities, Chinese medicine is again flourishing in its native land. Millions of Chinese depend mainly or solely on traditional herbal medicines, acupuncture, and related healthcare regimens for their primary medical care.

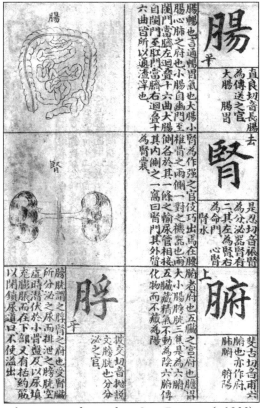

These images from a late Qing Dynasty (c.1900) dictionary reveal the influence of Western medical science on the Chinese conception of anatomy and physiology. Compare these with the more traditional images on p. 57.

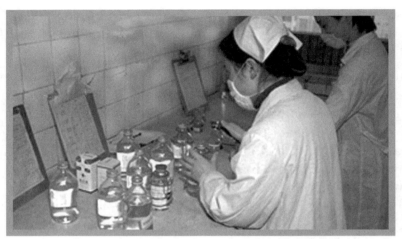

*Staff nurses for the in-patient ward ready herbal formulas
prepared as intravenous solution*

A vigorous movement has also developed towards integrated medicine in China as well as a World Medicine based on the integration of traditional and contemporary medical means. The compilation of the *Pharmacopoeia of the People's Republic of China* is guided by this principle.

As people throughout the world become increasingly interested and involved in using Chinese medicine, it is extremely important that the patterns of Chinese thought, research, and development be brought into clearer focus in the West. Our attempt to briefly summarize more than 2000 years of continuous development of medicine in China could not possibly be considered in any way complete. We hope only to offer readers a sense of the scope of its long history, and to establish the fact of its status as a well-developed, thoroughly researched, and valid tradition of medical science.

Granted that the nature of its centuries-old research and development differs in fundamental ways from the development of the scientific tradition in the Western world, it nevertheless reflects the special genius of the Chinese people. As Thomas Kuhn pointed out, "To understand it we shall need to know the special characteristics of the groups that create and use it." For if we fail to understand the cultural roots Chinese medicine, we cannot rationally expect them to survive and to endure in the effort to transplant Chinese medicine into Western soil. If, on the other hand, we can come to understand the special characteristics of Chinese medicine, we in the West can expect to enjoy the benefits of safe, affordable, and effective healthcare that Chinese medicine has to offer.

WHO CAN RIDE THE DRAGON?

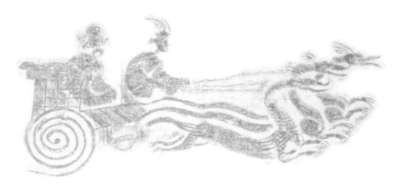

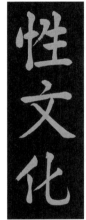

CHAPTER SIX

Sexual Culture, Longevity, and Immortality

Treasure your essence, nourish your shén, and take medicinal herbs. All these may lengthen your life, but if you do not follow the Dào of sex, none can truly benefit you.

—PENG ZHU, *SÙ NǙ JĪNG*

Present day civilization makes it plain that it will only permit sexual relationships on the basis of a solitary, indissoluble bond between one man and one woman, and that it does not like sexuality as a source of pleasure in its own right and is only prepared to tolerate it because there is so far no substitute for it as a means of propagating the human race.

—SIGMUND FREUD, *CIVILIZATION AND ITS DISCONTENTS*

MANY STEREOTYPES EXIST about the Chinese in Western minds. Like all stereotypes, the vast majority are inaccurate yet extremely durable. In particular, Chinese sexual culture has been vulnerable to stereotyping.

Worldwide, sexual stereotyping is an enormous industry; billions upon billions of dollars are spent every year developing and exploiting the manipulative power of sexual stereotypes. Putting this massive accumulation aside and looking directly at sex is a considerable challenge, charged as it is with the energy of life, yet contorted by the forces Freud and others have tried to illuminate. Sex, after all, is the means by which the race sustains itself. That generations continue to receive and transmit any tradition depends on the satisfaction of sexual drives without which humanity would simply cease to exist. Moreover, sexual identity forms a fundamental aspect of self-awareness as well as our social role. No sooner does a new life begin than it is associated with a powerful array of cultural stereotypes that match its gender: "It's a boy!" "It's a girl!"

With a characteristically pragmatic approach to sexuality in life and culture, the Chinese developed an extensive literature on sex, procreation, and intimate personal relationships. This is known as *fáng zhōng shù* or the "art of the bedroom." Among the various characteristics of these traditions, one notable feature emerges. The role of sexual life, as noted in the preceding quotation from Peng Zhu, who according to legend lived beyond the age of 800 years, was considered central to the achievement of health and longevity. Since the appearance of the oldest writings on the subject, cultivation of the bedroom arts has been understood as an integral aspect of the Chinese medical tradition.

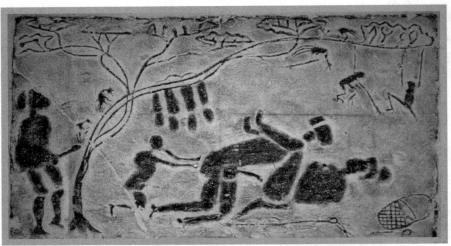

Rubbing of a Han Dynasty stone carving illustrating a theme from
The Book of Poems: "Under the Mulberry Tree"

In short, the Chinese have recognized since antiquity that to live to a ripe old age, we need to understand the role of sex and learn to manage our sexual drives. As such, the subject matter discussed in this chapter constitutes a subdiscipline of Chinese medicine. It summarizes a considerable body of literature and scholarship. This chapter offers an important perspective for understanding the traditional Chinese view of the human body and its fundamental substances and functions. The concerns of ancient writers evince a characteristic concentration on attaining longevity and maintaining health, wellbeing, and youthfulness. These concerns, as noted earlier, are typical of Chinese medicine in general.

性 What Is Chinese Sexual Culture?

For thousands of years the Chinese collected, studied, practiced, and passed on to posterity a tradition of knowledge and practice related to sex, reproduction, and the attainment of longevity and wisdom. Such material appears in the *Yellow Emperor's Canon of Internal Medicine* (*Huàng Dì Nèi Jīng*), the *Sù Nǚ Jīng,* Sun Si Miao's *Prescriptions Worth a Thousand Pieces of Gold* (*Qiān Jīn Fāng),* and numerous other ancient texts. Where the study of sex has only recently found its way into mainstream medical circles in the West, it has been a fundamental concern of Chinese medical experts for millennia. Medical scrolls discovered in 1973 at Ma Wang Dui in Changsha, Hunan Province were literally wrapped together with scrolls dealing with sexual cultivation. Certainly, at least since 168 B.C.E. when these scrolls were sealed inside King Ma's tomb, the Chinese arts of sex and healing have been closely linked.

For most of its recorded history, Chinese society has been male-dominated. Materials on sexual culture reflect this bias and are almost uniquely concerned with men's health, longevity, and the masculine attainment of wisdom through sexual practices, meditation, diet, and herbal therapy. There is nonetheless considerable attention paid to the sexual lives of women and the importance of sexual arousal and satisfaction for both the male and female partners. Not only is much valuable information available in these writings, they provide a unique perspective on the attitudes and concerns of medical theorists in the broad tradition of medicine in China. From the development of the arts of sexual cultivation we can trace the evolution of many concepts that directly migrated into traditional Chinese medical theory.

To understand and evaluate the material we present, we must first confront a number of basic issues. Questions of terminology are extremely important because many of the key words and phrases have double or triple meanings, not to mention vague and ill-defined ones. As with the vast majority of ancient Chinese medical texts, these materials were intended as blueprints or schematics to be interpreted and transmitted by direct personal instruction. Such instruction no doubt included clarification of the nomenclature.

The best and clearest example of the problems presented by the terms of sexual cultivation is one of the key concepts: *jīng* or "essence." In Chinese, this one word means both "essence" and "semen." As will become clear in reading the following translations, one of the primary concerns of the ancient theorists was the conservation and cultivation of sexual essence. In large part because of the homonymic characteristic of *jīng*, the material presents unique challenges to translators. As we described in the first chapter, Chinese words often have multiple meanings that coexist, forming a complicated mosaic of meaning. There are even cases where one or more of those meanings contradicts another. Sometimes context, syntax, and other purely linguistic cues decide which of several possible meanings should be stressed in translation. Regardless, the underlying vagueness remains. In the end, we must rely upon insight, and to some degree the intuition that derives from instruction and experience, to render such writings. Any English word chosen will obscure alternative renderings for readers unaware of this characteristic of the Chinese language.

"Essence" in Chinese medicine is an enormous concept. One of the three fundamental bodily treasures, *jīng, qì,* and *shén,* it is frequently discussed from many viewpoints and in relation to many medical issues. It is almost always related to the phenomena of reproduction, genetic endowment, sexual vitality, and longevity. The life-giving processes of nature are manifest in the concept of *jīng*. It can be understood as the sap of life, the irreducible essence that contains all the critical ingredients needed to make a new life that shares characteristics with its source. This is the *jīng* that plays so important a role in Chinese thought, the essence of Chinese sexual culture.

WHO CAN RIDE THE DRAGON?

房中水 TRADITIONS OF SEXUAL CULTURE IN ANCIENT CHINA

We often find that what first appears to be a homogeneous tradition is, on further investigation, a variegated blend of distinct patterns of thought and action. The martial arts, for example, are composed of many different schools, all featuring different approaches to the same basic questions. In the art of fighting it is easy to understand how different these traditions can be. Adherents of different schools literally come to blows to determine which way works best. With sexual cultivation, the problem of variety requires a different solution.

We have selected three major traditions of knowledge focusing on the subject of sex and, in particular, theories and practices for using sex to regulate health and promote longevity. Adherents of any one approach may contest the validity of any other approach to sexual culture. However, because our aim is to introduce the subject and illuminate its intimate relationship with Chinese medicine, we have chosen three representative forms.

黄帝 THE SEXUAL KNOWLEDGE OF THE YELLOW EMPEROR

Much of what we know of the legendary Yellow Emperor's approach to sexuality and sexual cultivation comes from an ancient source known as *Sù Nǚ Jīng*. Su Nu was one of five principal consorts who attended to his sexual life. Her name literally means "simple woman." Judging from the advice she gave her lord and master, she was far from ordinary. The ancient text that bears her name has been mostly lost over the course of centuries. Ye De Hui, a Qing Dynasty scholar, collected the available fragments and published a reconstituted version of this ancient manual of human sexuality. This edition stands today as the most complete presentation of this body of knowledge. Like many ancient texts, notably the *Yellow Emperor's Canon of Internal Medicine* and the *Classic of Difficult Issues*, the *Sù Nǚ Jīng* is presented as a series of dialogues between the Emperor and his consorts, mainly Su Nu herself.

The following passages from the *Sù Nǚ Jīng* illustrate the basics of this tradition of sexual cultivation and its role in achieving health and long life.

> The Yellow Emperor asked Su Nu, "My *qì* is weak and not in harmony. I always feel unhappy, as if I am in danger and cannot escape. What is happening to me?"

> Su Nu replied, "The reason this happens is that the *dào* of *yīn* and *yáng* are in disharmony and your sex life is not regulated. Usually women have more vitality than do men, just as water can overcome fire. One can organize this sexual life just as one controls the cooking of food: add just the right amount of water to regulate the fire, and the food will be delicious. Treat your sex life according to the theory of *yīn* and *yáng* and you can have all the happiness in the world. If you do not know these things, you will lose your life. How could one talk about happiness? How can we neglect our sex lives?

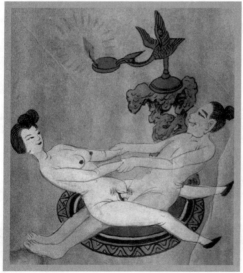

This image, as well as those on the following pages, is taken from a Qing Dynasty scroll depicting positions for sexual intercourse

Here we see the concern for an exhaustion of essence and its effects on the body and psyche. In fact, this became a central issue and a common concern for Chinese medical theorists, as is evident throughout the medical literature. The above passage from the *Sù Nǚ Jīng* reflects the notion of the kidneys as the storehouse of essence as well as the organ governing sexual potency.

The other key to its meaning is the metaphor relating *yīn* to *yáng*, water to fire, and man to woman. This pattern of interrelationships, this *dào* of *yīn* and *yáng*, is all-important in Chinese medicine. Here we see its expression in the art of sexual regulation:

> Su Nu said, "There is a girl named Cai Nu. She understands the *dào* of *yīn* and *yáng* [sexual matters] very well."

> The Yellow Emperor ordered her to pay a visit to Peng Zhu to inquire how to extend life and preserve health. When he was consulted, Peng Zhu answered thus: "To treasure one's *jīng* and nourish one's *shén*,

one can take many types of medicinals. This can produce longevity. But if one cannot understand the dào of sex, no matter how much medicine he takes, he still can not acquire the true benefit. When man and woman come together, it is just like heaven and earth creating each other. Heaven and earth have this way [dào] of intercourse; thus they live forever without limit. Human beings cannot understand or follow this dào of sex; thus they will harm themselves and die very quickly. If you fully understand the dào of yīn and yáng and can follow the right method of sex, then you are on the road to true longevity."

Here we again see an overriding concern for the harmonious conduct of one's sexual activities to "treasure one's *jīng* and nourish one's *shén.*" Peng Zhu was reputed to have lived for 800 years, not by relying on herbs alone but by paying attention to the importance of a healthy and well-regulated sexual life.

English speakers have developed an erroneous impression of Chinese medicine during the past twenty years. Acupuncture is probably the best-known and commonly accepted modality of the ancient Chinese systems of healing. Yet it is really what is called "herbal medicine" that is the central topic of traditional medicine in China. In these passages, it becomes clear that another more fundamental topic underlies even herbal medicine: sexual cultivation.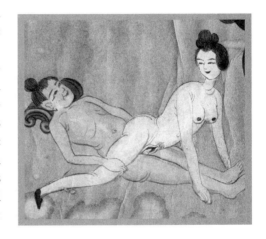

Cai Nu then bowed deeply to Peng Zhu and inquired, "Can I ask for more details of these matters?"

Peng Zhu replied, "The dào [method] of it is very simple and easy to understand. But people find it hard to trust and follow. Now the emperor works full time to rule and regulate the world. Of course he cannot deeply understand all aspects of the dào of preserving health. He is lucky that he has so many imperial concubines because he can follow the method of having sex with many young women while retaining his essence [semen]. This method will make one's body light and rid it of illness."

Sexual Culture, Longevity, and Immortality

In ancient China, there was a notable absence of sexual taboos. Instead, there is advice on how to become successful in sex. Sexual success, in the idealized terms stated in the preceding passage, included multiple partners, preferably young and beautiful women, at least for the Chinese elite who could afford them. Such ideals contradict traditional Western sexual mores. Whether or not such behavior exists in Western cultures, few Westerners today feel comfortable espousing a philosophy of sex that includes discussions of multiple adolescent partners.

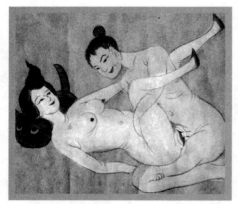

Regardless of the consequent tendency to obscure this aspect of Chinese sexual theory, these ancient Chinese ideas reflect a pragmatic, matter-of-fact attitude toward sex. Despite its contrast to changing sexual mores in the West, only a considered appreciation of Chinese thought and its understanding of men and women can help us fully comprehend Chinese sexual practices.

Su Nu said to the Yellow Emperor, "To have sex one should treat one's partner like tile and stone but treasure oneself like gold and jade. When the jīng is aroused, you should remove your penis from her body immediately. To have sex with a woman is like riding a horse with rotten reins; it is like approaching an abyss full of sharp knives. You fear falling into that abyss lest you lose your life. If one treasures one's essence life will be unlimited."

To "treat one's partner like tile and stone but treasure oneself like gold and jade" has a distinct meaning in Chinese literature. The idea is that one must safeguard against the loss of essence, and that this requires heightened self-awareness rather than a focus on one's sexual partner.

Clearly, in all the various theories and practices set forth by Su Nu and others, there is a theme of gathering qì or taking essence from one's sexual partner. This explains the explicit warning in the above passage. Sexual activity can be very risky, like "riding a horse with rotten reins": one is always in danger of losing control. On the other hand, treasuring essence "like gold or jade" will lead to health and long life.

The Yellow Emperor asked Su Nu, "What will happen if I now decide to refrain from sex for a period of time?"

Su Nu replied, "You cannot do this. Heaven and earth exhibit opening and closing. Yīn and yáng engage in intercourse to nourish and change. Human beings follow the method of yīn and yáng, governed by the changes of the four seasons to live their lives. If you now stop having sex, the qì of your essence could become diffuse; yīn and yáng would separate."

"How can one receive medicinal benefits from sex? One must practice a method of breathing and moving the qì within the body. Eliminate the old and breathe in fresh air: thus can one increase one's health."

"If the penis is not used in sex it will become like a snake turned to stone at the door of its lair from lack of movement. Thus one should constantly practice how to guide the qì to move throughout the body. This is known as dǎo yǐn. [The words mean to guide and lead]. Use the method of returning the essence to nourish the body. During sex one should arouse the jīng but not lose it. This is the Dào of Life."

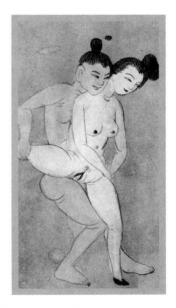

The *dǎo yǐn* referenced here is a practice of breathing and body movement, a variety of *qì gōng*. But the principal message of this passage is clear: abstinence will not help you to escape the dangers associated with sex. Only by carefully following the *dào* of sex can you eliminate the implicit dangers and achieve health and longevity.

The Yellow Emperor asked, "Then where are the limits to sex?"

Su Nu replied, "The dào of sex has its regulating principle: do not exhaust the man and the woman will be able to rid him of all illness. Both man and woman can enjoy the pleasure and increase each other's strength. But if you don't follow the dào of sex, your health will diminish day by day. In fact, the key point of the dào of sex is to calm the qì and pacify the heart to harmonize the mind. If these three are achieved, then the spirit takes command. The environment must not be too cold or too hot. To engage in sex, people should be neither too hungry nor too full. If these conditions are met, the movements will be naturally relaxed. When sexual intercourse begins, if one follows the principle of shallow penetration, in and out slowly and calmly, the woman will enjoy sexual pleasure and the man's vitality will increase."

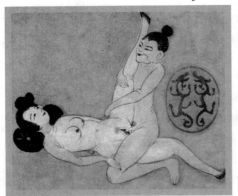

This passage clearly illustrates one of the key principles of this approach to sexual activity: regulation. To be sexually healthy, you must be able to moderate your sexual urges and regulate sexual conduct. In stark contrast to traditional Judaeo-Christian (and Islamic) attitudes toward sex, the aim of sexual discipline is to enhance pleasure rather than to eliminate it.

The Yellow Emperor asked Xuan Nu, "I've already understood the basic dào of yīn and yáng from Su Nu. However, I hope you can tell me more of the details."

Xuan Nu replied, "All things between heaven and earth are created by the intercourse of yīn and yáng. Yáng will transform [change, give birth] when it receives yīn. When yīn receives yáng, yīn will open and grow clearly. One yīn and one yáng must complement each other. Thus when the man senses that his penis will become hard, when the woman senses her vagina will open, then the two qì can have intercourse. The two jīng will open and begin to move and exchange."

"Men have eight limitations [prohibitions]. Women have nine regulations. If one does not follow these limitations, then the man will have carbuncles and the woman will suffer many diseases from her unregulated period. These things will result in the decrease of life; they will kill life. Follow the dào of yīn and yáng and sex will bring you only happiness. It will increase your life and make you healthy."

The Yellow Emperor asked, "What is the principle to follow in the practice of sex, the dào of yīn and yáng?"

Su Nu replied, "The way of sex has its principle which is to increase the man's qì and make the woman able to eliminate illness. It can also bring happiness to both man and woman, together with health and vitality. If one does not know the dào of sex, it will harm the health and result in increasing weakness.

"What is the dào of sex? It is to calm the emotions, harmonize the spirit and let the essence become interconnected. The environment cannot be too cold or warm. People should not feel hungry or full and should always be honest and upright; then the soul is free. At the beginning, the penis should move slowly and gently enter the vagina. It should move in and out slowly, not too much. This way will bring pleasure to the woman without exhausting the male."

The Yellow Emperor asked, "I want to have sex, but my penis cannot become hard. I feel so ashamed to face women. My sweat drops like pearls, but my mind desires sex. I use my hand to help my penis enter the woman but still cannot succeed. How can I get my penis hard? I want to know the dào."

Su Nu replied, "Your problem is very common among all men. To have sex with a woman there must be preparation. The man must harmonize his qì first. Then the penis will become hard naturally. If the man can follow the five constants [benevolence, justice, rites, faith, and wisdom], then the woman will have nine different reactions and five indications.

"When these signs appear, her body will be full of jīng qì. Now the man should use his mouth to take the woman's saliva. This [form of] jīng qì will transform within his body and arrive at the brain. This way will help avoid transgressing against the law of the Seven Damages [exhaustion of qì, leaking jīng, collapsed pulse, sunken qì, prolapse of organs, various stagnations, and exhaustion of blood], for it follows the way of the Eight Benefits [securing the jīng, stabilizing the qì, disinhibiting the organs, strengthening the bones, regulating the pulse, consolidating the blood, nourishing body fluids, and harmonizing the circulation]. This does not go against the Dào of the Five Ways. Thus the body can keep the beneficial qì within. How could one not eliminate any illness?

"If the five zàng and the six fǔ are healthy, then the outside will be full of light. The skin will be smooth and soft. The penis will become hard when you have sex no matter what time, and your strength will grow one hundred fold. It will be easy to overcome your partner. Where is the shame in that?"

孫 思 邈   SEXOLOGY ACCORDING TO SUN SI MIAO

In *Prescriptions Worth a Thousand Pieces of Gold (Qiān Jīn Fāng)*, Sun Si Miao, one of China's greatest doctors, carefully recorded the principles of focusing sexual activity to attain longevity. From a contemporary Western viewpoint, this material can seem starkly frank. It discusses various sexual techniques, the importance of sexual arousal, the role of the orgasm in health and wellbeing, and particularly the importance of conservation of the "vital essence."

Much of the material is best understood as an artifact of a culture that existed more than one thousand years ago. Sun Si Miao advises that, finances permitting, a man who seeks longevity should have many beautiful young women for his sexual pleasure. When understood in the context of Tang Dynasty China, this advice has rather different implications than it would in a contemporary context. Such disparities with modern cultural values notwithstanding, these materials describe a unique approach to the conservation and cultivation of sexual energies. It would be a shame and a great loss to discard or neglect such materials solely because they do not accord with contemporary morality. We quote here at length from Sun Si Miao:

> Theory says that most people below the age of forty will give way to their carnal desires, but when one reaches the age forty, he will suddenly feel the *qì* grow weak. Once the *qì* is weakened, one will be overcome with many different illnesses. If you do not take this seriously and do not take care to deal with it over a long period of time, it will completely overcome you. In the end, you will not be able to treat it.
>
> This is why Peng Zhu said, "Treat people with humane methods. Nourish the essence with essence." Thus when one reaches the age of forty, one must know the correct method of dealing with sex. The *dào* of sex is an intimate matter, yet few can follow it. The right way to engage in sex with ten women in one night is to prevent the loss of essence [not to ejaculate]. This is the aim of the study of sex. If this method is combined with the consistent ingestion of certain medicinals according to the change of the seasons, the *qì* and vitality will strengthen one hundred fold and wisdom will renew itself daily.

The purpose for my approaching the dào of sex is not to become a slave to carnality [i.e., not only to experience sexual enjoyment]. My purpose is to advise people to restrain themselves and preserve their health. The point is not to suggest that one take every opportunity to engage in sex with women to satisfy their lust. The real meaning of this study is to eliminate disease through sex. This is the principle of the study of sex. Thus some people who take medicines to increase their sex drive despite being below the age of forty will meet with disaster. One must be careful. Below age forty, one need not enter into discussions of the study of sex. For if one's sexual desire swells with lustful greed and he takes supplementing medicinals to increase sexual performance, the result will be exhaustion of the quintessential essence and lead one closer to death. Young men, especially, must be extremely careful of this. When reaching the age of forty, if one continuously takes dried powder of milk he can postpone aging. If one takes mica, in itself, it is enough to cure illness and extend life. After the age of forty, one should not take purgatives but rather take supplementing herbs.

In the past, the Yellow Emperor became godlike by having sex with twelve hundred women. Common people can come to their death as a result of sex with one woman. Knowing and not knowing are quite different. One who knows will only suffer from not having sex with enough women. The woman does not need to be extremely beautiful, but it is better if she is young and has not yet given birth and nursed a child. Her body should be full. If finances permit, one should select a woman with soft hair, bright eyes, a soft body with smooth skin, and a gentle voice. There should be ample flesh at every joint. The bones should not be big and wide. There should be no hair in the armpits or the pubic region. If there is hair, it should be soft and thin.

These requirements need not be strictly met. But if one engages in sex with a woman who has dry stiff hair, a dusky face, a neck shaped like a mallet with a prominent Adam's apple, a male-like voice and a big mouth, a high bridge of the nose and wheat-colored teeth, muddy eyes, hair growing on both upper and lower jaws, big wide joints, a thin body covered with yellow hair, and pubic hair that is thick and hard and all the hair growing against the natural grain, this will decrease the length of one's life.

The way to have sex is to wait until the *qì* is called and has arrived. The *yáng* is then aroused. One must proceed slowly. Play with the woman in the beginning to let the spirit and the mind intermingle long enough to summon the *yīn qì*. When the *yīn qì* surges forth, the penis will instantly become hard and strong. The man should go into action when his penis is hard. The movement should be slow and reserved. He must know to stop when certain movements occur. He must not throw himself into fast movements and strong motions. This will upset the five *zàng* organs and injure and harm both the pulse and the essence, leading to many types of illness. If one can engage in a lot of sex and keep in control of the motion, careful not to lose one's essence, all illness can be cured and life itself can be extended.

Follow this way and you will not stray from the heavenly path. You need not worry about how many women you have sex with. If you can have sex with 100 women and not deplete your essence; you will lengthen your life. Having sex with many women, you will have many chances to receive the female *qì*. The method for receiving *qì* from women is to put the penis deep inside of the vagina and sit still for a long time. Let the *qì* rise up. The face will become hot. Then use the mouth. Kiss the woman's mouth and draw forth the woman's *qì* and take it inside yourself. While doing this, the man can move his penis slightly, slowly. When certain motions are aroused, the movement should be stopped. The breath should be slow. The eyes should be closed.

If one can practice this sexual *qì gōng* one's strength will be increased. One will be able to have sex with more women, one after another. In order to gain the most benefit to one's health, a change of women is necessary. If one has sex with just one woman, the yīn *qì* will be depleted. The benefits of the yīn *qì* will be lost. The *dào* of yáng resembles fire. The *dào* of yīn resembles water. Water can overcome fire. Yīn can overcome yáng. To use one woman continuously will allow the yīn to overcome the yáng and decrease the yáng. Then what a man can get from a woman cannot make up for what he loses to her. But if one has sex with twelve different women and does not lose one's essence, aging will stop and more energy will develop. If one could have sex with ninety-three different women and retain one's essence he could live for ten thousand years!

A man lacking essence [semen] will easily fall ill. One with no essence will die. One cannot afford to ignore this. To engage in sex numerous times yet only release the semen once will increase the essence and protect one from vacuity. Conversely, if one has sex with just one woman yet releases his semen every time it will harm his health. The essence grows naturally and will replenish itself after being released in sex. But this happens slowly, little by little. It is not as fast and effective as having sex with lots of women while retaining the semen.

When people engage in sex they should breathe in through the nose and out through the mouth, slowly. One will naturally benefit from this kind of breathing. If there is a feeling like steam after sex, this is the phenomenon known as *dé qì* [to get or to take hold of the *qì*]. If one uses three *fēn* [0.3125 grams] of acorus powder mixed with ampelopsis powder, massaged into the body until the skin is dry, it will help the skin become strong and avoid damp sores. When one feels the semen about to release, close the mouth and open the eyes. Hold the breath and fold the hands into "baby's fists" [i.e., with the thumb held inside the other fingers, touching the middle joint of the middle finger]. Breathe in through the nose and circulate the *qì* throughout the body. Lying on the back, contract the lower part of the body and draw up the abdomen. Use the middle two fingers of the left hand to press the *cháng qiáng* [an acupoint in the perineum]. Then breathe out long and slowly, tapping the teeth a thousand times. This will lead the essence to nourish the brain. This will result in longevity.

If the essence is subject to rash actions it will damage the spirit. The *Classic of the Gods* says that the way to maintain youth is first to play with a woman sexually and then drink the jade liquid [which is produced]. The jade liquid refers to the saliva in the woman's mouth. Waken the sexual desire in both man and woman. Use the left hand. Keep the mind in the *dān tián*. There, inside, is "red *qì*." It consists of yellow within and white without. It goes through the transformations, becomes the sun and moon [of yīn and yáng] moving upward and downward within the *dān tián*. Then both enter into *ní wán*. The two come together and become one.

At this point one should retain the *qì*. Cultivate it. Do not breathe in or out. Through upper [the mouth] and lower [the genitals] the *qì* should be swallowed slowly. When certain motions are summoned and the semen is about to release, the man should withdraw immediately. An inferior man cannot perform this maneuver.

The *dān tián* is three *cùn* [roughly inches] below the navel. The *ní wán* is inside the head, directly behind the eyes. It appears as sun and moon in meditation. Its diameter appears to be three *cùn*. When the two [aspects] lose their shape and join together into one, it is known as "the sun eclipses the moon." Thus if in and out are subjected to the control of the mind, one's movements will be most beneficial.

It is also said that when a man and a woman practice the method of becoming gods [seeking immortality] through sex, they must take the *qì* deep inside and not allow the essence to be disturbed. In meditation the redness takes the shape of an egg inside beneath the navel. The movements should be gentle, both in and out. It [the penis] should be taken out when the essence has been called. A man who can manage this ten times in one day and not lose his essence will increase his life span. Both men and women can calm their mind together and meditate to increase their vitality through this method of cultivation. The method of regulating the essence according to the *Sù Nǚ Jīng* is to release the semen twice each month or twenty-four times per year.

If a man can do this he can live 200 years and still have good color in his face and be free of illness. If he also knows how to use the right herbs, he can get real longevity. When a man is in his twenties he can release the semen every four days. In his thirties he can release it once every eight days; in his forties, once every sixteen days; in his fifties, once every twenty days. In his sixties he should cherish his semen and not lose it to women. If a man is more than sixty yet still has good strength in his body, he can release his semen once each month. Those whose strength exceeds others should not hold back. If it accumulates with too much pressure, abscesses will result. If one's age exceeds sixty and he has not had sex for many months and still feels normal and calm, he should let the semen go naturally.

In the beginning years of Zheng Guan [a period in the early Tang Dynasty from 627-650 C.E.], I met an old man. He told me that lately he had felt the *yáng qì* surging forcefully in his body, rising up, filling him with sexual desire. This urge pressed him to have sex with his wife and they succeeded each time. He did not know whether he could do this at his age. Was it good or bad?

WHO CAN RIDE THE DRAGON?

I answered that this is a very bad sign. "Have you never heard of the oil lamp? When the oil in the lamp is almost depleted and the lamp is about to go out completely, it first begins to grow dark, then flares up brightly. But this spark of brightness must come to an end. Now, at your age you should have already retired from sex to store up your essence and calm your desire. Suddenly your sexual desire emerges. Can't you see this is not normal? I feel sorry for you. You should take good care of yourself."

Forty days later the old man took ill and died. This is the result of carelessness. Many people have a similar attitude. This old man is not alone; many others will go this same way. People who know how to preserve their health are careful to control their sexual desires when the yáng is full and rising. They do not give in to carnal desires as this slowly takes their life. Once you can control desire you can conserve the oil by turning down the light.

If you cannot achieve such control, if your desire runs free and you release your essence easily, it will be like the light from the oil lamp: it will always burn up the oil [i.e., it will be hard for you to protect your health]. I am afraid many people do not know this when they are young. Some may know but be incapable of believing until they get old and it is too late. It's difficult to treat disease. One should know it is late and take good care of oneself. One can still attain longevity and good health; thus there is nothing to disturb the mind. If you follow the dào of sex in your youth, it will help you cultivate your qì and remain on the road to immortality.

Su Nu posed a question: "Can one, being below age sixty, completely close the door and refrain from releasing his semen?"

Peng Zhu answered, "No! Man cannot live without woman. Woman cannot live without man. When a man lives without a woman, his mind becomes aroused. When the mind is thus aroused, the spirit will become exhausted. When the spirit is exhausted, it will shorten his life. If his mind is pure and rectified, it will assist him in attaining longevity. But people like this are rare, no more than one in ten thousand. If you merely repress your sexual urges they will become even harder to control, easily lost, and you will fall ill with leaking semen and turbid urine. This will develop into an illness known as `having sex with a ghost.' It will bring damage one hundred times over. There is an herbal formula to treat this disease."

The Yellow Emperor's prohibitions concerning sex say, "For people to have sex when angry, when the *qì* and blood are not calm will result in abscesses. To retain urine and engage in sex will cause painful urination and pain in the penis. To have sex when there is no color in the face, as when exhausted from a long journey, will damage the five *zàng* organs and cause them to be vacuous. This will result in the five impediments [impediment of the heart, liver, spleen, lung, or kidney that result from insufficiencies of yīn, yáng, *qì*, and blood of the organ]. This will also affect one's ability to produce children. To have sex with a woman whose period has not completed will result in vitiligo in the man. Mercury must not come in contact with the sexual organs. The grease from deer and pigs can cause impotence."

These notions can appear archaic, obscure, even irrelevant. They can best be understood in their historical and cultural context. More than a thousand years ago, Sun Si Miao applied himself to the study and refinement of what was then already an ancient tradition of magic and medicine. In his time, civilization in China flourished and the cultivation of life became a widespread preoccupation of Chinese nobility and intellectuals. They sought with the knowledge and resources they had at their disposal to synthesize theories and methods to prolong life and increase their enjoyment of it.

Sun Si Miao's work is pivotal in the development of Chinese medical theory. His writing provides one of the clearest iterations of the principles of yīn and yáng as they relate to sexuality and health. His work as an alchemist brought Chinese medicine to new heights as he labored to incorporate the essence of ancient lore into a systematic method of refining medicinal herbs and minerals into effective preparations.

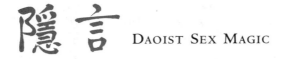 DAOIST SEX MAGIC

Daoist alchemists sought to retard the aging process and prolong life. Two methods were used. One involved the development of formulas and techniques to synthesize medicinal herbs and minerals that might be ingested to attain this goal. The other involved the cultivation and control of the intrinsic "treasures" of the body through meditation.

WHO CAN RIDE THE DRAGON?

The ultimate aim of this second category, however, was not merely longevity but immortality. Theories and techniques of Daoist sexual cultivation fall mainly into this second category, the search for the "internal elixir." This sexual magic aimed at refinement of the "essence" which began with not releasing it during intercourse. By following the methods prescribed for breathing and circulating the *qì,* one stored essence which was then converted into spirit. Through these practices the Daoist initiate strove to become an immortal.

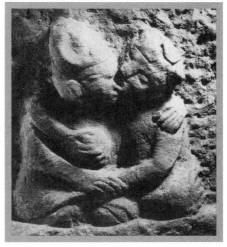

Stone carving of a couple in a Daoist sexual embrace

The Daoist approach to immortality stands in sharp contrast to that of Western religions. In Judaism, Islam, and Christianity, for example, believers put their faith in an almighty God and trust that through devoted obedience to divinely-given codes of conduct they will be rewarded with eternal life. The Daoists viewed the matter personally and directly. They believed that through a variety of methods, all based on similar principles, they could transform the body's essential substances; in effect, transform the body itself. This transformation has been described in many ways, but never as something that occurred after death. It was a transformation that took place during life and that precluded death, a transformation that embodied the essence of life. They sought this transformation through drugs, through breathing and exercise, and through sexual cultivation and refinement of the "essence."

We put the word "essence" in quotations here to underscore the importance and scope of this term in understanding the material in the lengthy quotation that follows (see p. 189), which is translated from the Ming Dynasty text, *Xìng Mìng Guī Zhǐ,* a book that was given to us by a Daoist monk on Qing Cheng Mountain outside our home in Chengdu, Sichuan Province. One day while visiting this fellow at the temple that stands on the summit of Green City Mountain, we asked him what someone who wished to study the Dào should do. He stopped in midstep and smiled at us. "There is a book that anyone who wants to follow the Dào should read first." *Xìng Mìng Guī Zhǐ* is the book he gave us later that day.

Where the *Xìng Mìng Guī Zhǐ* quotation that follows is almost solely focused on the attainment of immortality through sex from the viewpoint of the male partner, there is also much information in the text that relates to female sexual practices. To be sure, China of the Ming period was a male-dominated society. Modern readers who can look beyond the surface may be able to see material that is relevant to their own experience, regardless of its possible conflicts with contemporary sensibilities.

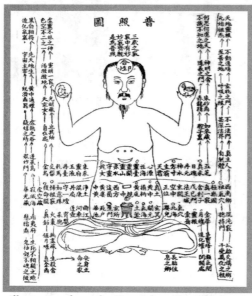

Illustration from the Xìng Mìng Guī Zhǐ showing the spiritual root of heaven and earth in the body

There is no better place to focus such a search for implicit meanings than on the meaning of yīn and yáng. Although the literature displays a definite male bias, the substance of yīn-yáng theory is curiously free of such prejudice, for yīn and yáng solely and only co-exist. In their constant interplay one rises and one falls, but neither can sustain a superior position permanently. Indeed, they are understood to be complementary forces, the yáng impelling and sustaining yīn, the yīn containing and restraining yáng, so that in their harmony they support life itself.

This implicate order of yīn and yáng is reflected in Chinese folklore by the fact that among immortals, women are more or less equally well represented as men. The status of Su Nu illustrates this fact. Not only was she the Yellow Emperor's consort, she was his teacher. Her yīn essence provided him with substantive notions that allowed him to consolidate his vital yáng and achieve immortality.

Thus we see that despite cultural values which reflect an atmosphere of male dominance, ideologically such material contains the germ of sexual harmony. This harmony was understood to be a dynamic rather than a static condition. In their conduct throughout the multidimensional exchanges which take place during sexual intercourse, both men and women find direction through the pattern of ideas contained within the theory of yīn and yáng.

WHO CAN RIDE THE DRAGON?

One primary focus, again perhaps the result of the male-dominant attitude of the writers of *Xìng Mìng Guī Zhī*, is the concentration of attention on retaining "essence." *Jīng* is critically important to the practice of Daoist sex magic. As noted earlier, "essence" is one of the words used in English to translate *jīng*. Like so many Chinese words, *jīng* has many meanings. Two of these meanings are essential to understanding *jīng* in Daoist sexual writings. As we have already discussed, the first is "essence" and the second is "semen." The word develops its complete meaning through the harmonic interaction of "essence" and "semen" which can, and often should, be simultaneously understood. The word *jīng* in Daoist sexual writings is used to refer to both the concept of essence and to the substance of seminal ejaculation.

The problem that develops as a result of this interaction is that it is often not clear when advice concerning retention of *jīng* refers to withholding or preventing male ejaculation and when it concerns something more difficult to grasp. This "something," which is indeed more difficult to grasp, is the concept of retention of essence itself. Many writers have resolved this problem by formulating a general prohibition against the release of semen in intercourse. We do not seek to purvey either the same or a contradictory understanding. Rather, we want to emphasize that the text of the *Xìng Mìng Guī Zhī* contains an ambiguity that cannot be resolved unless readers search for deeper understanding by reference to other texts and their innate understanding of their own bodies and their natural rhythms.

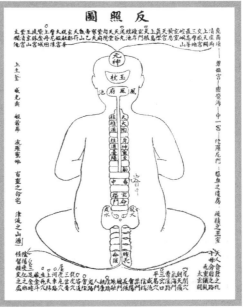

Illustration from the Xìng Mìng Guī Zhī showing the principal acupoints through which the qì circulates

The ancestral spiritual aperture closes to gather congenital essence: Lao Zi calls it xuán pìn zhī mén [the gateway to the Mysterious Female]. The Daoist says the Mysterious Female is the place to cultivate the Golden Elixir. The whole procedure of cultivation from beginning to transformation of the spirit takes place in this location. Thus, if one knows where this orifice is, he can attain the Dào of the Golden Elixir.

What is the ancestral aperture and where is it? Ancient Daoists had many ways of explaining it, calling it by different names, for example: host of the congenital essence; ruler of the ten thousand manifestations; the basis of tài jí, the root of chaos [the primordial state of the universe]; the land of perfection; the place of condensation; the valley of emptiness; the source of all creation, and so forth. It is hard to list all the names that have been given.

This orifice is not the mouth, nose, heart, kidney, liver, spine, lung. Nor does it lie between the two kidneys. It is not in the dān tián [One cùn (inch) and three fēn (one tenth of a cùn) below the navel] nor in ní wán [the acupoint at the apex of the skull] nor in qì hái [an acupoint on the lower abdomen].

The great Daoist Chun Yang used the theory of life to explain it, saying, "when the father and mother begin to have sex, the mysterious light of the ancestral streams into the mother's womb. It has the shape of a ball filled with brightness that shines." Confucians called it rén. It is also known as wú jí. Buddhists call it a pearl. As well, it is known as the "bright circle."

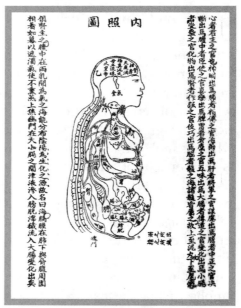

Illustration from the Xīng Mìng Guī Zhǐ showing the systematic correspondence of the principal organs and their functions

In Daoism it is called dān [elixir] and líng guāng [mysterious spiritual light]. Yet all these names are given to this one qì of the orifice, the supreme essence of the Great Chaos. It is the origin of the created body, and marks the beginning of the receiving of qì. It is the basis of life and the ancestor of the ten thousand transformations. When the act of sex has come to its end, the jīng and the blood coalesce and cover the outside [of this ball].

WHO CAN RIDE THE DRAGON?

This becomes what Confucius termed tài jí. The five zàng and six fǔ organs, the four extremities, the hundreds of bones, all take shape because of this. Thus can one see, hear, stand upright and walk; all because of this. One can give and receive humanity, justice, the rites, and wisdom because of this. And one can become a sage, a god, versed in correct conduct, literary and martial arts [from this phenomenon].

Thus the basic origins all come from tài jí. Cān Tóng Qì [an important Daoist text, from the Eastern Han Dynasty 25–220 C.E.] says, "Man's body originally comes from emptiness. The primordial essence sprays like clouds due to the force of qì. The Mysterious Female comes into being as this qì condenses. It creates the path of wisdom at the upper position [ní wán]) and the sea of qì at the lower position [dān tián]. The mind and intelligence, one's nature, are contained in this pass of intelligence. There also are contained one's life, qì, and destiny. Although life separates into the Dragon [male] and the Tiger [female], the root of life is controlled in the ancestral aperture." Thus Lao Zi says, "The door of the Mysterious Female is the root of heaven and earth."

This excerpt details the Daoist objective of creating and cultivating the internal elixir. The next chapter specifically addresses the sexual act and its importance in this process.

The Yì Jīng says, "when the qì of yīn and yáng unite, joining heaven and earth, the ten thousand transformations result. When male and female engage in sexual intercourse, the ten thousand creatures appear on earth. Heaven and earth give birth to all creatures through the mixture of yīn and yáng. Thus does the medicine take shape for the internal elixir by means of sexual intercourse between yīn and yáng. There is no creation that can take shape without the mixture of yīn and yáng."

The paramount importance of the union in the process of creating this internal elixir is underscored in the following passage.

If the qì of heaven and earth do not come together, the dew will not appear. If the qì of the tiger [male] and the dragon [female] do not come together then the seed of the true One will not come to creation. Once this seed of the true One does exist, what is the way to grasp and congeal the golden elixir?

The meaning of the next passage is not as clear and depends on an understanding of the *Yì Jīng* trigrams [see Chapter 4].

> *Sexual intercourse of Tiger and Dragon is the method of reuniting the three elements. By rejoining Heaven* ☰ *and Earth* ☷ *you mix yīn and yáng, embrace nature and life, to return the two to One. Thus when a man and his wife have sex, they enter the void in a trance. Together they absorb one another's qì. Their movements linger. The two qì mix and interact like heaven and earth. They come together and mix their seeds for all things to take shape and find form. It is like the light of the sun mixing with the light of the moon to shine together. It circles the Ancestral Aperture. It forms the qì of origin [the qì that is not separated into yīn and yáng] and becomes the essence, the great original, the true One. This is the original root of the great medicine. It is the basis of the creation of the elixir.*

There is much that is unclear in these passages. Yet one thing does emerge. For the Daoist, the act of sexual intercourse was a seminal step in an alchemical process that not only explained and participated in the ongoing regeneration of the human race, but formed the basis of a magical act meant to extend life indefinitely. There can be no question that Daoist sensibility beheld sex as the emblem as well as the wellspring of life's creation. This applied to the creation of the new being as a result of sex as well as the creation of this abstracted fraction, the Golden Elixir.

To quote Joseph Needham, writing on a separate yet related topic, "This is a great theme, which deserves better justice than can be done it within the framework of such a book as this." The "book" he was referring to was his extensive, multivolume work, *Science and Civilisation in China.*"

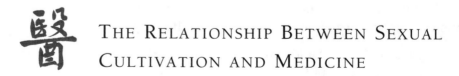 ## THE RELATIONSHIP BETWEEN SEXUAL CULTIVATION AND MEDICINE

We end this brief look at Daoist sexual magic with something that is well within the scope of this book, that in fact lies at the essence of this book: the relationship between sexual cultivation and Chinese medicine.

The relationship between the study and practice of sexual cultivation and medicine and health is to some extent self-evident because of the shared terms and concepts. Many people are intuitively aware that sex and health are linked without holding to a specific theory of how or why. In the West, the widespread acceptance of sex as a topic for medical study can be traced to the work of Sigmund Freud. Freud considered repression of the sexual drive a cause of mental disorders. As a rough comparison between the Western attitude and the traditional Chinese point of view, we can say that the ancient Chinese theorists simply did not stop with mental problems. They viewed proper sexual functioning as integral to health and considered it a usual and proper subject of investigation when health gave way to disease.

This understanding came into medical theory largely through the Daoist philosophy of harmonizing with nature. Rather than advocating the restraint of sexual desire, the Daoists studied and practiced how to harmonize and direct sexuality to improve human health and wellbeing. This attitude is reflected in the Chinese medical understanding of sexuality. Just as significantly, however, this frank and careful long-term study of human sexuality revealed valuable information that guided medical theorists and clinicians throughout the centuries, increasing their understanding and ability to intervene therapeutically in the complex interrelationship between their patients' sexual lives and their medical condition.

There is no clearer manifestation of yīn and yáng than in the interrelationships between man and woman. It is indeed only through the interplay of yīn and yáng (taking yīn to stand for Woman and yáng to stand for Man) that the human world continues. Thus, the sexual act can be understood as both the fundamental and the ultimate emblem for life force, qì. Since its very beginnings, Chinese medicine has been concerned with how to nurture and foster the growth and development of this life force.

Taken in these terms, it becomes easy to see that the study of sex, the cultivation of sexual energies through the conscious management of sexual practices, and virtually all issues related to sex were (and continue to be) inextricably bound with the pursuit of wellbeing. This has led to the development of both sexual techniques for treating disease as well as sexual "exercises" to be practiced by those who seek to strengthen their constitution, cultivate their intrinsic energies, and enhance their lives. To such efforts, the Daoists appended the ultimate aim of their naturalistic metaphysics: immortality.

Living forever may or may not be an aim to which we aspire in the modern world. Yet contemporary people are turning to such ancient sources of wisdom for a better understanding of issues that affect not only the length but the quality of their lives. One thing that our exploration of such material has taught us is that an absolute prerequisite to successful study and eventual understanding is a thorough familiarity with the basic concepts, terms, and phrases of the subject. Thus we return to the language of Chinese medicine.

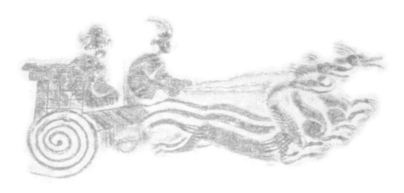

CHAPTER SEVEN

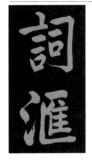

Key Terms of Chinese Medicine

THIS BOOK ENDS more or less where it began: with a detailed look at the concepts of Chinese medicine as each is understood in the Chinese language. By so doing we hope to merge the ideas expressed in the preceding chapters with an understanding of these key terms. Those who can ride the dragon—our metaphor for comprehending the principles of Chinese medicine—are those who understand its concepts in the Chinese frame of reference. We offer this annotated list of terms hoping that it will stimulate discussion, debate, understanding, and ultimately a more informed use of the words, ideas, and precepts of Chinese medicine.

Our goal is not the creation of definitive explanations or a translational standard. Although translational standards must exist, their creation is simply not our aim. Our aim is to introduce and illuminate the problems facing those who seek to define and use such standards.

Therefore, to facilitate clear communication between patients, their doctors and insurance companies, HMOs and other healthcare organizations—in fact anywhere Chinese medicine is studied and applied—we offer the following discussions. Hopefully these will be become part of an ongoing process to cultivate a better understanding of these concepts and to utilize them more effectively.

術 語 THE TAXONOMY
OF THE NOMENCLATURE

If you have ever reviewed a Chinese-language dictionary of Chinese medical terms, you will have probably noticed a categorical arrangement. The taxonomy of Chinese medical nomenclature reflects the subject's underlying theoretical structure. Typically, books on the subject begin with a discussion of basic theoretical principles: yīn-yáng and five phases. From here they proceed to fundamental structural terms (i.e. physiology and anatomy) such as: zàng fǔ and jīng luò. The next category typically consists of basic diagnostic terms: pathogenic factors, therapeutic methods, and so forth.

It is important to recognize that this traditional arrangement is itself a piece of wisdom concerning not just the pedagogy of Chinese medicine, but also its development. To deviate from this classical arrangement is to discard an important element; therefore, the words presented below are not arranged alphabetically nor according to any other convention more familiar to the Western reader.

This format presents a view of the body as an aggregate of universal forces and substances. Among these, three emerge as fundamental "treasures." They are jīng, qì, and shén. In another light, the whole body, in fact all of creation, can be understood in traditional Chinese terms as an accumulation of qì. When the qì gathers, life begins. When the qì disperses, life ends.

The arrangement of the nomenclature can thus be understood as a tool that has developed over thousands of years to help those who seek to understand the movements and other behaviors of this mysterious, life-sustaining qì. Herein we have preserved the basic arrangements found in most Chinese texts, hoping to make this book more useful to those working to advance their knowledge and understanding through study of many of the books that are available.

RETHINKING THE TRADITIONAL CATEGORIES OF CHINESE MEDICAL NOMENCLATURE

To those unfamiliar with the structure of Chinese medical theories, the Chinese arrangement of medical terms often seems strange and confusing. Light can be shed on this subject by comparing the arrangement of materials in textbooks. When we examine the contents of a typical textbook of anatomy in Western science, we discover that the materials are arranged in a supposedly organic pattern that reflects (and continues to perpetuate) a particular view, a specific understanding of the human body, what it is, what it does, and how it works. The conventional paradigm of the body is so well established that the entire subject of gross anatomy is considered "complete." It is recorded and institutionalized as such in textbooks. More importantly it is generally accepted by theorists, researchers, clinicians, and the public at large to be the only accurate expression of truth about the body. Thus, when we encounter paradigms from other contexts or other cultures, we find them odd, unfounded in scientific fact, and consequently judge them to be invalid.

The traditional Chinese image of the body and its various dynamic systems and subsystems is substantially different from that of Western medical science. The Western anatomist sees the body as a hierarchy of structure and function, just as his textbooks present it. To understand the body in these terms, we must first understand the whole schematic. It is arranged in terms of progressively more complex systems beginning with single cells through colonies of cells, embryonic structures, tissues, organs, and systems, up to and including the entire organism, the individual human life. The particular data imparted to medical students on the pages of their textbooks conforms to this overriding structure, and material that does not fit that organization is discarded.

An example is the idea of the *jīng luò* in Chinese medicine. Where does this concept fit within the Western anatomist's model of the body? The answer to this question is problematic because the *jīng luò* do not fit neatly into the Western paradigm, and cannot be observed with biomedical instruments. Western anatomists do not see them, so they do not "exist."

The ancient Chinese were far more interested in how things functioned and particularly how they interacted; for example, how stimulating one part of the body—a finger or toe—could produce remarkable effects in distal regions—the abdomen or lower limbs. They sought to perceive and comprehend the nature as well as the basic pattern of these complex relationships. The sense of anatomy and physiology that they developed after thousands of years of such investigation was therefore far more concerned with patterns of acquisition, consolidation, utilization, and function of *qì* than of organic structure.

Early illustrators of the body sought to depict their sense of how the universal *qì* circulated throughout and thus animated the body, gave rise to the mind, and produced and influenced the emotions and all the organic functions of the body. These ancient cartographers of the body's essential substances and activities succeeded in producing an eloquent, dynamic description of patterns by which the information needed to function was communicated from one part of the body to another. Their systematic chart was complete and all-integrating, providing anyone who could read and understand it with a blueprint of how the organism functioned. With this knowledge, diagnosis and treatment of disease could proceed by interpreting and correcting disharmonies in the body's patterns of propagating information, *qì*.

This is a distinctly different sort of chore than determining where to make an incision to remove a gallbladder. It requires a different mind-set, a different attitude towards life, and a different set of tools, the most basic of which are, naturally, the words by which we understand all other concepts and tools.

It says a great deal about Chinese medicine that most of its dictionaries begin with a section devoted to the words and terms that describe and define yīn and yáng. Yīn and yáng are truly the root of all medical theory and practice in China. When you compare this profoundly philosophic root to its opposite in Western medical science, you confront what might be fairly called the first and greatest of the cultural gaps between these two disparate forms of medicine.

There is simply no corresponding philosophical concept or structure at the root of Western medical science. It may well be argued that like Chinese medicine, medicine in the West can trace its roots to ancient, primitive forms and practices. Historians can demonstrate philosophical and philological correspondences between modern medical science and alchemy, or the medical arts of the ancient Greeks. However, few if any textbooks of medicine begin with these discussions. Hardly a word is uttered about the importance or even the existence of such connections

Who Can Ride the Dragon?

in the halls of medical science. The simple fact is that whatever vestiges of such a philosophical root may exist, they do not form the foundation of any contemporary medical practice. Medical students are trained to keep up with the latest, most modern research and methodology, and the most profound statements of authority begin with the words, "The latest research indicates …"

Modern medicine always strives to be just that: modern. Newness, improvement, and progress seem inextricably intertwined: what is newest is surely the best. Here again, we see the power of cultural influences on medical thinking. Clearly, this influence has not always wisely guided the development and deployment of Western medicine. Thalidomide was once the "newest and the best." Antibiotics were long considered the prize of biomedicine, and new antibiotics were praised, year after year, for their disease-destroying capabilities. Recently, researchers began to recognize that each successive generation of "newer and better" antibiotics was not simply curing patients but facilitating mutated or resistant strains of "super-bugs" that could survive the antibiotic onslaught. Typically, the response of Western medical researchers has been to intensify their efforts to develop new antibiotics.

Chinese medicine, quite to the contrary, places enormous emphasis on honoring the traditions of its antiquity. By placing ancient materials at the entrance of the subject, Chinese medical writers demonstrate their understanding that it takes time for concepts about the body, the nature of disease, and suitable, sustainable approaches to treatment to prove themselves safe and effective. We have tried to preserve this flavor of the traditional in the list that follows, while paying due attention to the background of Western readers.

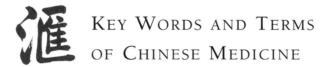 # KEY WORDS AND TERMS OF CHINESE MEDICINE

In the sections that follow we present more than one hundred of the basic terms of Chinese medicine. The words are arranged according to traditional categories that begin with fundamental concepts and proceed to areas of specialization. They are translated and accompanied by brief explanations and interpretations. As we have stated elsewhere, we have not attempted to offer standard technical definitions for the terms. The aim of this section is to present an overview of the basic terminology of the subject, to discuss the various meanings of these basic terms, and to offer readers pathways for understanding other Chinese medical terms that they may encounter.

A Note on Dictionaries

To let readers know what we had in mind in compiling this list of words and meanings, we offer the following brief discussion of dictionaries. Although it is not our aim to present a dictionary in the sense that dictionaries have come to be known, any compilation of words and their meanings can be understood to be a dictionary of sorts. The model we adopted in preparing the material for this section follows an older version.

Prior to the mid-nineteenth century, English-language dictionaries were quite different than they are today. The turning point in English lexicography spans fifty years from 1869 to 1919. The defining element in this drama of definitions is the *Oxford English Dictionary*. Conceived as an effort to crystallize the perfection of language that mid-nineteenth century English in London was believed to be, and to proof it against the vagaries of time and change, the "O.E.D.," as it has come to be called, succeeded in ways that its original authors and editors might never have conceived.

There is scarcely a dictionary available in the English language today that does not mirror the basic conceptual infrastructure of the *O.E.D.* Briefly, this infrastructure can be understood as the application of Darwinian "organicism" to philology. If humankind was the product of evolution, so therefore must various languages also be evolving systems of meaning and communication. Philologists reasoned that there must have been a proto-language from which all others evolved, and despite the non-existence of a single word from this supposed proto-language, an entire vocabulary was developed to serve as the roots of modern languages. This was the common wisdom of the day in which the *O.E.D.* was conceived, and this is the indelible impression it has left on the English language.

The *O.E.D.* puts the work that follows in perspective and emphasizes the differences between our model and the generally accepted notion of a dictionary today. One good example of the model we have employed is Samuel Johnson's *Dictionary of the English Language*. Published in 1755, Dr. Johnson's "dictionary of the English language in which the words are

deduced from their originals and illustrated in their different significa-
tions by examples from the best writers" was a milestone in the art of
lexicography. Johnson himself was quick to note what a thankless art his
was, by including the following lines at the very beginning of his preface:

> *It is the fate of those who toil at the lower employments of life to be
> rather driven by the fear of evil than attracted by the prospect of
> good; to be exposed to censure, without hope of praise; to be dis-
> graced by miscarriage, or punished for neglect, where success would
> have been without applause and diligence without reward. Among
> these unhappy mortals is the writer of dictionaries whom mankind
> have considered not as the pupil but the slave of science.*

Johnson's dictionary, a massive work that filled two volumes, stood
as the paradigm of English lexicography for one hundred years or more.
It was certainly not the first but it was the best English language dictionary until the *O.E.D.* Lacking the guidance of the comprehensive, scientific structure that the *O.E.D.*'s lexicographers synthesized for use in their
work, Johnson proceeded in an eclectic fashion, gathering words, meanings, and illustrative uses from the great writers of the English language.

He also inserted much of his own opinion, and indeed his own igno-
rance, into his dictionary. In more than one place he states, "I don't
know," as the description of words for which he failed to find an adequate
meaning. Along with such personal information, Johnson's work also
reflects the society, the attitudes, and thought of his day. One clear example of such revelation can be seen in the definition of the word "oats." We
quote it below in its entirety as it appears in the definitive 4th edition.

> *Oats. N. [axen, Saxon] A grain, which in England is generally
> given to horses, but in Scotland supports the people. It is of the grass
> leaved tribe; the flowers have no petals, and are disposed in a loose
> panicle: the grain is eatable.*
>
> *—The meal makes tolerable good bread.*   *—*MILLER
>
> *—The oats have eaten the horses.*   *—*SHAKESPEARE
>
> *—It is bare mechanism, no otherwise produced than the turning of
> a wild oatbeard, by the insinuation of the particles of moisture.*
>   *—*LOCKE
>
> *—For your lean cattle, fodder them with barley straw first, and the
> oat straw last.*   *—*MORTIMER'S HUSBANDRY
>
> *—His horse's allowance of oats and beans was greater than the
> journey required.*   *—*SWIFT

In our own approach to providing readers with the meanings of the words that follow, we have employed, if not Dr. Johnson's wit, at least his attitude and at the very least his reliance upon others to illustrate either typical or important uses. We hope that you will benefit from this method of study and that it will help you gain deeper understanding and insight into the original nature of the terms.

The following definitions often begin with excerpts or quotations taken from *A Practical Dictionary of Chinese Medicine* (Second Edition, Paradigm Publications, 1998), which presents the most coherent compilation of a translation standard available to date. To these definitions we have appended additional comments as needed to help clarify both the literal and figurative meanings of the words and terms. We have also provided quotations from earlier authors of Chinese medical literature, so as to provide readers with a further sense of how these terms have been used. This approach is intended to develop a sense of the many layers of meaning which exist beneath the surfaces of virtually the entire nomenclature of Chinese medicine.

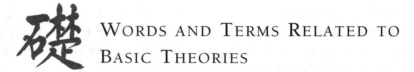

WORDS AND TERMS RELATED TO BASIC THEORIES

The theories of Chinese medicine are based on underlying philosophical, cosmological, and ontological concepts and precepts that have been developing in China for thousands of years. There are several key terms used to discuss these most fundamental principles. Many of these words have been introduced and discussed at varying length in the text. The word *qì* appears in numerous places in the foregoing chapters and in the following list, reflecting its pervasive presence in the mind/heart of Chinese medicine.

Qì

The motive force or impetus for all processes of change and transformation in the universe. The word *qì* has several meanings. (See below and Chapter 1 for further discussions of this idea.) The concept of *qì* in Chinese medicine originally came from ancient philosophical sources. It evolved into medical theories and practices to explain human physiology and pathology. From a philosophical or cosmological perspective, *qì* is the substantive origin of the whole universe. It is the basic "substance" from which everything on earth is constituted. As noted elsewhere, Zhuang Zi wrote, "Throughout the world there is only one *qì*." In Chinese medicine, *qì* is the basic substance that constitutes the human body. The relationship between the philosophical meaning of *qì* and the medical meaning can be clearly seen in these quotes:

—*Qì: 1. Air, gas, vapor, flatus (e.g., Belching of Putrid Qì). 2. Smell. 3. Aura. 4. Environmental forces (e.g., Cold; Dampness, Dryness, etc.). 5. Nature (e.g., the Four Qì). 6. Any of various dynamic phenomena of the body (e.g., Source Qì; Construction Qì; Bowel and Visceral Qì; Channel Qì).*

A PRACTICAL DICTIONARY OF CHINESE MEDICINE

—*The life of a human being is the gathering of qì. When qì gathers together, life comes forth. When the qì disperses, life ends in death.*

ZHUANG ZI

—*The qì of heaven and earth engage in intercourse, thus creating human beings.*

SÙ WÈN, THE YELLOW EMPEROR'S CANON OF INTERNAL MEDICINE

—*Mankind is born of the qì of heaven and earth and grows according to the laws of the four seasons.*

SÙ WÈN, THE YELLOW EMPEROR'S CANON OF INTERNAL MEDICINE

—*Heaven nourishes man with five (distinct forms of) qì. Earth nourishes man with the five flavors. The five qì enter through the nose and are stored in the heart and lungs. They illuminate in five colors on the face and resound clearly in the voice. The five flavors enter through the mouth and store in the stomach and intestines. The essence extracted from the five flavors nourishes the five qì. When the qì is in harmony it produces body fluids and saliva. This gives rise to spirit (shén, q.v.).*

SÙ WÈN, THE YELLOW EMPEROR'S CANON OF INTERNAL MEDICINE

—*Qì is the basis of man.*

NÁN JĪNG, THE CLASSIC OF DIFFICULT ISSUES

Wú jí

Infinity, infinite, limitlessness; a term from Daoist metaphysics referring to the state or condition of existence prior to the differentiation of yīn and yáng. In the context of Daoist philosophy, *wú jí* is used as part of the explanation for how all life came to be. Recall the line from the *Dào Dé Jīng* which reduces this entire sequence of being into simple if perplexing terms:

> *Dào gives birth to one; One gives birth to Two;*
> *Two gives birth to Three; Three gives birth to all things.*

In this sense, *wú jí* can be understood to represent One. It is symbolized by a circle. Yet even this Oneness is understood to come about as the result of a process—the grand process, that is, the process that embraces all others, known as *dào*. The beginning of this great process is known as "emptiness."

Another term for the state of unity existing in emptiness is *tài yī*. The concept of *tài yī* can be understood as the beginning of nothingness. The transition point from nothing to something is described as the moment at which the *qì* began to vibrate. In other words, the great void began to open and close. In this cosmological sequence there follows a great change, *tài yī*. This great change is the change from static to dynamic force. The result is the differentiation of yīn and yáng, and from the resulting interplay of yīn and yáng, all life, all things, and all existence. This is the *yī* of the *Yì Jīng*.

This dynamic state of existence is symbolized as *tài jí*. *Wú jí* is understood to represent the state of completeness prior to *tài jí* (yīn and yáng) in this cosmological sequence. The word *wú* means "no, not, none, without, absence of, negation." The word *jí* means limit, pole, extreme, boundary, border.

> —*Know the bright. Keep to the dull. Be a guide to the world. To be*
> *a guide to the world, follow your innate nature without straying and*
> *return to wú jí.*
>
> DÀO DÉ JĪNG

Tài jí

The grand ultimate; extreme limit; referring to the essential reduction of all matter, energy, space, and time to their irreducible components, yīn and yáng. *Tài jí* is the state or condition of existence that proceeds from *wú jí*. *Tài jí* can thus be understood as the unity resulting from the "two-ness" of existence. The word *tài* means "great, utmost, too much, extreme." The word *jí* means "limit, boundary, extent."

—*Tài jí comes from wú jí and is the mother of yīn and yáng.*

TÀI JÍ QUÁN LÙN OF WANG SONG YUE, AS TRANSCRIBED BY LI YI YUD

—*One qì began to separate. The truth dominates and carries forth its own judgment. It is self-reflective, filled with respect and solemn silence. Yīn and yáng sentenced to separation. This is tài jí. This is the Two (One gives birth to Two). This is called the sovereign void. In this sequence of existence, when the universe developed to the stage represented by tài jí, it had reached the beginning of life. The light of intelligence (líng guāng) found shape to compose.*

Tài jí has but one logic. In motion it is called Time. It takes but one breath, although this breath lasts the whole universe. Condensed, it is the size of millet. Yet it contains the whole universe. It is called the True Seed. To liberate and return to the root, to ease the breath and disappear into another world: this is the 'time of tài jí.' To become pregnant with this seed and harvest the fruit, to have sex and be pregnant with child, these are the True Seed. If one can protect the two extremes (jí) and not lose them, one can prolong life beyond the length bestowed by heaven.

XÌNG MÌNG GUĪ ZHĪ

—*Yì [the Yì Jīng] has tài jí. Tài jí gives birth to the two primordial forces. These two forces give birth to the four seasons. The four seasons give birth to the eight trigrams.*

BOOK OF CHANGES

Yīn-Yáng

Two complementary opposites that together comprise the essential elements of all phenomena and events in the whole universe. The concept of yīn and yáng forms an evolutionary step in the cosmological sequence developed in ancient Chinese philosophy. In the development of these words, we see important aspects of the growth of the naturalistic philosophy that became most closely associated with Daoism. Originally, the two words were meant to differentiate between sides of a hill. *Yīn* meant the north side or shady side; *yáng* meant the south side or sunlit side. In the earliest dictionary of the Chinese language, *Shuo Wen Jie Zhi*, from the period of the Eastern Han, the two words were explained as: "Yáng: high, bright. Yīn: dark, the north side of the mountain or south side of the river." The *Yì Jīng* says: "One yīn and one yáng form the *Dào*." The terms were used to explain all natural phenomena from the alternation of day and night to the intricate structures and functions of the human body.

> —*Two mutually complementary and opposing principles in Chinese thought; one dark, female, receptive (yīn), and the other bright, male, active (yáng). The two principles categorize phenomena of like quality and relationship. The Chinese characters denoting yīn and yáng denote the dark side and light side of a mountain respectively, i.e., light and darkness. Many other phenomena are closely related to light and dark.*
>
> *For example, light is associated with heat, and darkness is associated with cold. Daytime is the warm, bright part of the day; nighttime is the cold, dark part of the day. Summer is the season of greatest light and heat; winter is the season of greatest darkness and cold. South is the position of greatest light and heat; north is the position of greatest darkness and cold. Daytime and summer are the times of activity; nighttime and winter are times of rest and quiescence. The upper and outer aspect of an object tends to receive sunlight; the inner and lower aspects of objects tend to be dark. Light (yáng) is to darkness (yīn) as heat is to cold, as day is to night, as summer is to winter, as north is to south, and as activity is to rest. Hence heat, daytime, summer, south, and activity are yáng, while cold, night, winter, north, quiescence are yīn.*
>
> A PRACTICAL DICTIONARY OF CHINESE MEDICINE

Wŭ xíng

1. The five phases (through which matter cycles in its unending circulation throughout all material substances); hence, 2. The five phases: metal, water, wood, fire, and earth. This phrase refers to a theoretical structure that supports much of traditional Chinese thought. It is as an

WHO CAN RIDE THE DRAGON?

extension or expression of yīn-yáng theory applied to the nature of material substance and to the various interrelationships that exist between matter in its different phases. These five phases function metaphorically, providing images which ancient theorists employed to organize their thinking about the physical world. The word *wǔ* means five. The word *xíng* means "passage, pathway, route, to go, all right."

—*The five phases, like yīn and yáng, are categories of quality and relationship. The ancient Chinese saw phenomena within the universe as the products of the movement and mutation of five entities: wood, fire, earth, metal, and water. These represent qualities that relate to each other in specific ways. Other groups of five phenomena that have like qualities and relate to each other in analogous ways are said to belong to the five phases.*

A PRACTICAL DICTIONARY OF CHINESE MEDICINE

—*The ancestral rulers forged the world from metal, wood, water, fire, and earth.*

GUÓ YǓ

Sì shí

The four seasons; a general term for spring, summer, autumn and winter in which the third month of summer (the sixth month of the Chinese lunar year) is termed "long summer." The four seasons are correlated with the five phases thus: spring–wood; summer–fire; long summer–earth; autumn–metal; winter–water. There are also alternate views of their relationships. One such view places the earth phase in each season, coming at its end, in the same position in which it stands in long summer in the sequence given above. Thus, the third month of spring is correlated with the earth phase, as is the third month of summer and each of the other seasons. This relationship is expressed in the following passage from the *Classic of Categorizations* written in 1624 by Zhang Jie Bing:

—*The spleen belongs to the Earth which pertains to the center in its influence and manifests for eighteen days at the end of each of the four seasons. Thus it does not pertain to any season on its own.*

ZHANG JIE BING, THE CLASSIC OF CATEGORIZATIONS

In Chinese medicine, the four seasons are considered to be primary aspects of etiology and pathology. Understanding seasonal changes and the proper methods to employ to adjust the body accordingly became essential aspects of medical theory and practice. The entire second chapter of the *Yellow Emperor's Canon of Internal Medicine* is devoted to this topic.

> —*Thus the four seasons and yīn and yáng are the root of everything in creation. Hence the Sage conceives, develops, and nourishes yáng in spring and summer, yīn in autumn and winter to follow the root. In this way, the sage, along with everything in creation, maintains himself at the gate of life and growth. Those who rebel against the root sever their own root and ruin their true selves. Yīn and yáng and the four seasons are the beginning and the end of everything and the cause of life and death. Those who disobey this natural law will give rise to calamities and visitations, while those who follow the law of the universe remain free from dangerous illness, for they are the ones who have attained the Dào.*
>
> YELLOW EMPEROR'S CANON OF INTERNAL MEDICINE, VEITH TRANSLATION

The word *sì* means "four." The word *shí* means "time, season."

> —*Mankind and heaven are connected and involved in one another. The pulse must follow the change of the four seasons.*
>
> YĪ XUÉ XĪNG WÙ

> —*Mankind was born of the intercourse of the qì of heaven and earth. Thus there came about the law of the four seasons to maintain life.*
>
> SÙ WÈN, THE YELLOW EMPEROR'S CANON OF INTERNAL MEDICINE

 # WORDS AND TERMS RELATED TO THE STRUCTURE AND FUNCTION OF THE BODY

The following words can be understood as the terminology of traditional Chinese anatomy and physiology. They describe the body in terms of its component parts, paying particular attention to its functional and relational organization.

WHO CAN RIDE THE DRAGON?

1. Refined substance; the refined and life-supporting substance flowing in the body. 2. Vital transformative potential, particularly as expressed in the functional forces of the various organs, tissues, and systems of the body. (See p. 202 for further discussion.)

1. Congenital essence; the fundamental substances constituting the body. 2. Acquired essence of food; fundamental substances capable of maintaining vital activities. 3. Reproductive essence, sperm or ovum.

The word *jīng* has a variety of meanings and all are related through the concept of "essence." These include: "refined, selected; essence, extract; perfect, excellent; meticulous, fine, precise; smart, sharp, clever; energy, spirit; skilled, conversant; sperm, semen, seed; goblin, demon, spirit; the essence of life, the fundamental substance which maintains the functioning of the body."

> —*That which is responsible for growth, development, and repro-duction, and determines the strength of the constitution, and is manifest physically in the male in the form of semen. Essence is composed of earlier heaven essence (congenital essence), which is inherited from the parents and constantly supplemented by later heaven essence (acquired essence) produced from food by the stom-ach and spleen. Later heaven essence is considered to be the same as, or a derivative of, the essence of grain and water from which qì, blood, and fluids are also produced. Essence is often referred to as essential qì, and because it is stored by the kidney, it is also called kidney essential qì.*

A PRACTICAL DICTIONARY OF CHINESE MEDICINE

> —*Jīng is the origin of the body.*

SŪ WÈN, THE YELLOW EMPEROR'S CANON OF INTERNAL MEDICINE

> —*Jīng is the beginning of man's life.*

LÍNG SHŪ, THE YELLOW EMPEROR'S CANON OF INTERNAL MEDICINE

> —*Jīng and qì provide nourishment for one another. As the qì gath-ers, the jīng becomes plentiful. If the jīng is plentiful, the qì will*

prosper. If one exhausts one's jīng, it will result in weakness of qì and invite illness. Such illness poses grave danger to one's health. Thus the jīng is the greatest treasure of man's life.

LÍNG SHŪ, THE YELLOW EMPEROR'S CANON OF INTERNAL MEDICINE

Shén

1. Spirit; a general term for vital activities especially as reflected in the external appearance of the internal (physiological and/or psychological) condition of the body. As such, it is the primary criterion for diagnosis and prognosis. 2. Mind; referring to thought and the state of consciousness. 3. The law of nature, that is, the substantive movements and changes in the natural world. 4. Dominant aspect, that is, chief commander of jīng and qì and all vital activities. 5. Marvelous, mysterious, godlike, god.

The word *shén* refers to the eternal dimension of life, to the magical or heavenly aspects of being alive. It means, "god, deity, divinity or divine nature; supernatural; magical; expression, look, appearance; smart, clever."

—*(In a wider sense) that which is said to present in individuals with healthy complexion, bright eyes, erect bearing, physical agility, and clear coherent speech. It is said, "If the patient is spirited, he is fundamentally healthy; if he is spiritless, he is doomed." Thus, the spirit sheds useful light on the severity of a given complaint.*

A PRACTICAL DICTIONARY OF CHINESE MEDICINE

—*Shén is the foundation of heaven and earth. It is the great beginning of all things on earth.*

SHUŌ YUÁN

—*Exhausting the qì will cause the shén to vanish.*

DŌNG YĪ BǍO JIÀN

—*If one cultivates one's jīng and shén, illness can not invade.*

SÙ WÈN, THE YELLOW EMPEROR'S CANON OF INTERNAL MEDICINE

—*The heart is the monarch of all the organs; from it the mysterious brightness of the spirit (shén) comes forth.*

SÙ WÈN, THE YELLOW EMPEROR'S CANON OF INTERNAL MEDICINE

WHO CAN RIDE THE DRAGON?

—The shén is the ruler of the whole body. It controls the seven affects. Harming the shén will result in illness.

DŌNG YĪ BǍO JIÀN

—If you have shén, you will progress towards health. If you lose your shén, you lose your life.

SÙ WÈN, THE YELLOW EMPEROR'S CANON OF INTERNAL MEDICINE

Xuè

Blood; an essential component of the body derived from the refined foodstuff that is consumed and made assimilable through the processes of digestion and metabolism. It is the liquid substance that circulates in the blood vessels to deliver nourishment to all parts of the body.

The word *xuè* is used to mean the blood itself in the same sense as it is understood in modern physiology. It is also used to mean something specific to Chinese medicine: the substantial fraction of the circulatory system in a unique relationship with the circulation of *qì*. The clearest expression of this unique relationship is found in the *Yellow Emperor's Canon of Internal Medicine*: "The blood is the mother of *qì*; the *qì* is the commander of the blood."

—The red fluid of the body that according to traditional explanations is derived from the essential qì derived from food by the stomach and spleen, which becomes red blood after being transformed by construction qì and the lung. Blood flows to all parts of the body, and is governed by the heart. By the action of the heart and lung, it flows through the vessels, carrying nourishment to the whole of the body. All the bowels and viscera and all parts of the body rely on the blood for nourishment. The heart and liver are said to have their own blood, the terms "heart blood" and "liver blood" meaning blood in relation to the functions of those two viscera.

A PRACTICAL DICTIONARY OF CHINESE MEDICINE

—The middle jiāo receives the qì, extracts it [from food] and turns it into red blood.

LÍNG SHŪ, THE YELLOW EMPEROR'S CANON OF INTERNAL MEDICINE

—The function of the blood is to nourish.

NÁN JĪNG, THE CLASSIC OF DIFFICULT ISSUES

—If the blood and vessels are in harmony and healthy, the jīng and shén will abide within.

LÍNG SHŪ, THE YELLOW EMPEROR'S CANON OF INTERNAL MEDICINE

Yíng

Construction (*qì*), constructive nutriment; one of the essential substances for sustaining vital activities. It is derived from the digested food and absorbed by the internal organs. It circulates through the channels as a fraction of the blood to nourish all parts of the body. It is the essential ingredient of the blood, and is responsible for the production of blood and the nourishment of body tissues. The blood and the *yíng* are inseparable. Thus they are often referred to as *yíng xuè*. The word *yíng* has a variety of meanings, including, "seek; operate (as in the operation of a business); camp, encampment, barracks; battalion (i.e. subdivisions of military organization)."

—An abbreviation for construction qì, which is an essential qì formed from the essence of food and which flows in the vessels. Construction is considered to be an aspect of the blood. ... The English construction conveys the original sense of the yíng in the medical context, reflecting the analogy to national administration, in which construction or maintenance of infrastructures (the various parts of the body) is paired with defense.

A PRACTICAL DICTIONARY OF CHINESE MEDICINE

—Yíng is the jīng qì of food. It harmonizes and nourishes the five zàng organs and irrigates the six fǔ organs. It enters the blood vessels, following the channels upward and downward throughout the five zàng and connects the six fǔ.

SÙ WÈN, THE YELLOW EMPEROR'S CANON OF INTERNAL MEDICINE

—Yíng qì extracts itself (from food) and becomes the blood, entering the vessels to nourish the four limbs, the five zàng, and the six fǔ.

LÍNG SHŪ, THE YELLOW EMPEROR'S CANON OF INTERNAL MEDICINE

Wèi qì

An aspect of *qì* that functions to defend the body at the level of the skin and muscles. It flows outside the channels and blood vessels, forming a "defensive force" that defends the body from exogenous evils. It also functions to regulate the secretion of sweat. The word *wèi* means "defend, external protection, safeguard."

> —*A* qì *described as being "fierce, bold, and uninhibited," unable to be contained by the vessels and therefore flowing outside them. In the chest and abdomen it warms the organs, whereas in the exterior it flows through the skin and flesh, regulates the opening and closing of the interstices (i.e., the sweat glands ducts), and keeps the skin lustrous and healthy, thereby protecting the fleshy exterior and preventing the invasion of external evils.*
>
> A PRACTICAL DICTIONARY OF CHINESE MEDICINE

> —*The function of* wèi qì *is to bring warmth to the boundary (of the body). It replenishes the skin, nourishes the skin's surface and controls the opening and closing of the pores.*
>
> LÍNG SHŪ, THE YELLOW EMPEROR'S CANON OF INTERNAL MEDICINE

Jīn yè

Fluids; a general term for all the liquid components of the body other than the blood. It is one of the basic substances that transforms into blood. It exists extensively within the human body, between organs and tissues serving a nutritive function. It is composed of two categorically different substances that form a single entity and can transform one into the other. These are:

Jīn, liquid, or thinner fluids. These have the function of nourishing the muscles and moisturizing the skin. The *jīn* also permeates the blood vessels and thus nourishes the blood. The sweat and urine originate in thin fluids. They have greater mobility and motility than the *yè*, humor, or thicker fluids [see below] and belong to *yáng*.

Yè, the thicker fluids. These function to nourish the bones and the internal organs, brain, and marrow. They also moisturize the apertures of organs and the joints. Having greater density or substance but less mobility and motility, they are understood to belong to the yīn category.

In general, *jīn* and *yè* share a common nature. They are both derived from the essence of food. They influence one another and transform into one another as they circulate throughout the body, cyclically nourishing the entire organism. Thus they are generally referenced together as *jīn yè*. The word *jīn* means "ferry, crossing, ford; saliva; sweat; moist, damp." The word *yè* means "liquid, juice, fluid."

> —*The term "fluids" embraces all the normal fluid substances of the human body. The term refers to fluids actually flowing within the human body and to sweat, saliva, stomach juices, urine, and other fluids secreted by or discharged from the body. The main functions of fluids are to keep the bowels and viscera, the flesh, the skin, the hair, and the orifices adequately moistened, to lubricate the joints, and to nourish the brain, marrow, and bones. Though referring to a single entity, "fluids" is often differentiated into two basic forms, liquid and humor, to highlight specific characteristics. Liquid refers to fluid that is relatively thin, mobile, and yáng in quality, whereas humor denotes thicker, less mobile yīn fluid.*
>
> A PRACTICAL DICTIONARY OF CHINESE MEDICINE

> —*Jīn and yè have their own distinct passageways. The jīn passes through the triple burner and transforms to qì, bringing warmth to the membranes between the skin and the muscles and nourishing the skin. The yè will not travel thus.*
>
> LÍNG SHŪ, THE YELLOW EMPEROR'S CANON OF INTERNAL MEDICINE

> —*When the pores open, the perspiration emerges from the jīn. When the food enters, the qì is replenished. The essence moistens the bones. It enriches the brain and marrow, and smoothes the skin. This is the yè.*
>
> LÍNG SHŪ, THE YELLOW EMPEROR'S CANON OF INTERNAL MEDICINE

Wŭ zàng

The five viscera; the so-called "solid" organs. This is a name given collectively to the heart, liver, spleen, lungs, and kidneys. These organs constitute one category that is distinguished from the six *fŭ* organs [see below] in both structure and function. The *zàng* organs are thought of as solid, essence-containing organs. (Recall that the concepts and terminology relating to the internal organs in traditional Chinese medicine differ considerably from those of modern Western medicine.) The word *zàng* means "viscera, internal organ."

> —*Organs of the chest and abdomen. The five viscera are the heart, lung, spleen, liver, and kidney. The pericardium is considered a sixth viscus in channel theory. The six bowels (paired by functional relationship with the viscera respectively) are the stomach, small intestine, large intestine, gallbladder, bladder, and triple burner. The function of the viscera is to produce and store essence, that of the bowels is to decompose food and convey waste.*
>
> A PRACTICAL DICTIONARY OF CHINESE MEDICINE

> —*The function of the wŭ zàng is to store the jīng qì and not release it. Thus they can be substantial but not filled.*
>
> SÙ WÈN, THE YELLOW EMPEROR'S CANON OF INTERNAL MEDICINE

> —*When the jīng qì is full this is called substantial. When the body is full of food, this is called filled. The function of the wŭ zàng is to store jīng qì. Thus they can be substantial but not filled.*
>
> WANG BING'S COMMENTARY ON THE SÙ WÈN

> —*The wŭ zàng are for storing jīng, shén, xuè, qì, and the soul.*
>
> LÍNG SHŪ, THE YELLOW EMPEROR'S CANON OF INTERNAL MEDICINE

Lìu fŭ

The six bowels; the six "hollow" organs; a term given collectively to the gallbladder, stomach, large intestine, small intestine, urinary bladder, and the hard-to-define "triple burner" (*sān jiāo*). In contrast to the five *zàng* organs, the six *fŭ* organs are considered to be hollow and to be involved in the transportation of substances rather than the storing of essential substances. The word *lìu* means "six." The word *fŭ* means "bowel." Like *zàng*, it is a special term of Chinese medicine. From the Tang to the Qing Dynasty it was the word used to designate the political subdivision commonly translated as "prefecture." Its sense is a division of space, especially such a division meant for containing or housing.

—The liù fŭ function to transport food but do not store. Thus they can be full but are not substantial. When food enters through the mouth it fills the stomach but not the intestines. When it passes from the stomach, the intestines become full as the stomach empties.

SÙ WÈN, THE YELLOW EMPEROR'S CANON OF INTERNAL MEDICINE

Qí héng zhī fú

Literally, "extraordinary organs"; this is a designation given to a group of organs that resemble the *fŭ* organs in structure and the *zàng* organs in function, including the bones, blood vessels, gallbladder, and uterus. The brain and the marrow are also placed in this category. The word *qí* means "strange, queer, rare; surprise, wonder, astonish." The word *héng* means "permanent, long lasting; perseverance; normal, usual, common; constant." *Qí héng* means "extraordinary." The word *zhī* is a particle in this case denoting the adjectival function of *qí héng*.

—Any of a class of organs comprising the brain, the marrow, the bones, the vessels, the uterus, and the gallbladder, distinguished from the bowels on the grounds that they do not decompose food and convey waste and from the viscera on the grounds they do not produce and store essence. The gallbladder is an exception, because it is classed both as a bowel and as an extraordinary organ. It is considered a bowel because it plays a role in the processing and conveyance of food, and stands in interior-exterior relationship with its paired viscus, the liver. However, the bile that it produces is regarded as a "clear fluid" rather than as waste; hence it is also classed among the extraordinary organs.

A PRACTICAL DICTIONARY OF CHINESE MEDICINE

—The brain, marrow, bone, blood vessels, gallbladder, and womb are born of the qì of the earth. They represent the nature of earth and belong to yīn. Thus they can store essence and not release it. They are called qí héng zhī fú.

SÙ WÈN, THE YELLOW EMPEROR'S CANON OF INTERNAL MEDICINE

WHO CAN RIDE THE DRAGON?

Jīng luò

The channels and network vessels or meridian system forming an essential feature of the human body. The *jīng luò* comprises the network of routes for the circulation of *qì* and blood. Through this network the entire body is interconnected: the viscera, bowels, the extremities, upper and lower, interior and exterior, left and right—in short, all parts of the body—are thus brought into communication with each other. The *jīng luò* joins the tissues and organs of the body together into an organic whole. The word *jīng* means "warp; channels; longitude; manage; constant, regular; scripture, canon, classic; menses; pass through; as a result of; stand; bear." The word *luò* means "something that resembles a net; the subsidiary channels; to hold something in place with a net; to wind or twine."

> —*The pathways of blood and qì pervading the whole the body, connecting the bowels and viscera, the limbs and joints. The channels are the main pathways of qì and blood, whereas the network vessels are smaller branches ensuring supply of qì and blood to all localities. Disturbances in the channels are reflected in abnormalities along their course. Acupuncture, acupressure, and cupping are largely based on the theory of the channels and network vessels.*
>
> A Practical Dictionary of Chinese Medicine

> —*The word jīng means main path. The tributaries of the jīng extend and are called luò.*
>
> Entrance to the Study of Medicine

> —*The jīng luò belong to the zàng fǔ and connect with the limbs and joints on the exterior.*
>
> Líng Shū, The Yellow Emperor's Canon of Internal Medicine

Mài

1. Vessel; a channel through which blood and *qì* flow. 2. The pulse and its condition. *Mài* is a medical word that means "arteries and veins; pulse; vein."

> —*Any pathway of the blood or of qì.*
>
> A Practical Dictionary of Chinese Medicine

The heart controls the mài, and the mài house the shén.

Líng Shū, The Yellow Emperor's Canon of Internal Medicine

Shū xué; Xué wèi

Acupoint; the general name given to those locations that lie along the *jīng luò* that possess particular qualities and functions. (See Chapter One for a fuller explanation and description of the words *shū* and *xué*.) *Wèi* means "place; location."

> *A place on the surface of the body where qì and blood of the channels and network vessels gather or pass. Through the channels and network vessels, points are connected to other parts of the body and notably the bowels and viscera, whose state of health they can reflect. Various stimuli such as needling, moxibustion, massage, acupressure, and electroacupuncture can be applied at points to regulate internal functions.*

> A Practical Dictionary of Chinese Medicine

> *The Yellow Emperor said, "I've heard there are 365 acupoints to symbolize the days of the year."*

> Sù Wèn, The Yellow Emperor's Canon of Internal Medicine

Dān tián

The site three *cùn* (approximately one and one third inches) below the navel and approximately one-third of the distance from the navel to the spine. In ancient Daoist texts there was often mention of three *dān tián*. For example:

> *The brain is the sea of marrow which is the upper dān tián. The heart is the crimson palace that is the middle dān tián. The site three cùn below the navel is the lower dān tián. This lower dān tián is the mansion in which to store jīng. The middle dān tián is the mansion for storing qì. The upper dān tián is the mansion for storing shén.*

> The Heavenly Classic

Daoist beliefs and practices related to these locations in the body stem from a fundamental conviction that human life was endowed with superior *qì* from heaven and earth. This endowment takes the form of *jīng, qì, shén*. The *shén* is born from the *qì*, and the *qì* is born from the *jīng*. Thus in Daoist practices aimed at prolonging life, the *dān tián* are the positions for the concentration of these three "treasures." The name given to this process of storage, concentration, and refinement was "internal elixir." The word *dān* originally meant the color red. Because of its color, cinnabar (mercury, an ingredient used in herbal medicine) came to be known as *dān*. This word was also used to refer to the small red pellets or pills made from cinnabar and other ingredients which were intended by Daoist alchemists to aid in the process of cultivating the internal elixir. Thus the word *dān* also came to mean "internal elixir." The word *tián* means "field, farmland, crop land."

> 1. An area three body-inches (cùn) below the umbilicus, believed by Daoists to be the chamber of essence (semen) in males and the uterus in females. 2. Any of three mustering positions in qì gōng, including the lower cinnabar field (xià dān tián) located below the umbilicus, the middle cinnabar field (zhōng dān tián) located in the pit of the stomach (scrobiculus cordis), and the upper cinnabar field (shàng dān tián) located in the center of the brow.

A PRACTICAL DICTIONARY OF CHINESE MEDICINE

> —The dān tián is positioned three cùn below the navel. Its diameter is four cùn.

NÁN JĪNG, THE CLASSIC OF DIFFICULT ISSUES

Sì hǎi: *suǐ hǎi, xuè hǎi, qì hǎi, shuǐ gǔ zhī hǎi*

The word *hǎi* means "sea, ocean." It is often seen in the names of acupuncture points generally referring to a class of points where the *qì* behaves as if converging like water in the sea. *Suǐ* means "marrow." *Shuǐ* means "water." *Gǔ* means "grain." The four seas; a term applied collectively to *suǐ hǎi*, the sea of marrow, referring to the brain where the marrow is seen to converge; to *xuè hǎi*, the sea of blood, referring to a) the *chōng mài* (thoroughfare vessel, one of the eight extraordinary vessels) where the blood of all the channels is seen to converge; b) the liver, where the blood is stored; c) an acupoint on the spleen meridian located above the knee; to *qì hǎi*, the sea of *qì*, referring to a) an acupuncture point named *dàn zhōng* at the level of the nipples in the center of the chest where *qì* originates and converges (also known as *shàng qì hǎi*, "upper sea of *qì*"); b) the *dān tián*, the site three *cùn* below the navel (also known as *xià qì hǎi*, "lower sea of *qì*"); and c) an acupuncture point on the *rèn mài* (controller vessel), located on the anterior midline of the body approximately one and a half inches below the navel; and to *shuǐ gǔ zhī hǎi*, the sea of water and grain, referring to the stomach where the food is received and stored.

> —The Magic Pivot states, "People have four seas ... the sea of marrow, the sea of blood, the sea of qì, and the sea of grain and water. ... The stomach is the sea of grain and water. ... The thoroughfare (chōng) vessel is the sea of the twelve channels. ... Chest center is the sea of qì. ... The brain is the sea of marrow."

> The four seas can be regulated at specific points on the body: the sea of marrow at *bǎi huì* [GV-20, Hundred Convergences] and *fēng fǔ* [GV-16, Wind Mansion]; the sea of qì above and below the pillar bone [collar bone] and at *rén yíng* [ST-9, Man's Prognosis]; the sea of grain and water at *qì chōng* [ST-30, Qì Thoroughfare] and *zú sān lǐ* [ST-36, Leg Three Li]; and the sea of blood at *dà zhù* [BL-11, Great Shuttle], *shàng jù xū* [ST-37, Upper Great Hollow] and *xià jù xū* [ST-39, Lower Great Hollow].

A PRACTICAL DICTIONARY OF CHINESE MEDICINE

> —All the marrow belong to the brain.

SÙ WÈN, THE YELLOW EMPEROR'S CANON OF INTERNAL MEDICINE

> —The brain is the sea of marrow.

LÍNG SHŪ, THE YELLOW EMPEROR'S CANON OF INTERNAL MEDICINE

> —The qì gathers and accumulates in the chest in the place known as the sea of qì

LÍNG SHŪ, THE YELLOW EMPEROR'S CANON OF INTERNAL MEDICINE

> —Humans extract qì from food. The stomach is the place that receives food, thus the stomach is the sea of food and water.

LÍNG SHŪ, THE YELLOW EMPEROR'S CANON OF INTERNAL MEDICINE

WHO CAN RIDE THE DRAGON?

The gate of life; referring to a location on the back between the two kidneys. The kidneys are considered to be the storehouse of the *jīng* and therefore the source of *qì* in the body. Early medical theorists envisioned this location between the two kidneys as the seat of *yáng* and therefore the gate of life. This *yáng* is sometimes considered as heat or fire. *Mìng mén* fire is associated with the primary fire of the heart in an assistant capacity. Modern research has produced evidence correlating the ancient Chinese concept of this region of the body with the physiological role and importance of the adrenal cortex and the various adrenocortical mechanisms and responses.

The word *mìng* means "life; fate, destiny; order, command." The word *mén* means "door or gate."

> —*The term "life gate" first appears in the Inner Canon (Nèi Jīng) where it refers to the eyes. Reference to a "life gate" as an internal organ body first appears in the Classic of Difficult Issues (Nàn Jīng) which states, "The two kidneys are not both kidneys. The left one is the kidney, and the right is the life gate." The question of the life gate invited little discussion until the Ming and the Qing, when various different theories were put forward: a) both kidneys contain the life gate; b) the space between the kidneys is the life gate; c) the life gate is the stirring qì between the kidneys; d) the life gate is the root of original qì and the house of fire and water; e) the life gate is the fire of earlier heaven or the true yáng of the whole body; f) the life gate is the gate of birth, i.e., in women the birth gate and in men the essence gate.*

A PRACTICAL DICTIONARY OF CHINESE MEDICINE

> —*Mìng mén (the gate of life) is the basis of the five zàng organs.*

SÙ WÈN, THE YELLOW EMPEROR'S CANON OF INTERNAL MEDICINE

> —*Mìng mén is the active qì between the two kidneys. It is not fire or water. It is the pivot of life, the root of yīn and yáng.*

YĪ ZHĪ XŪ YÚ

Qī qiào

The seven orifices; the clear orifices, the orifices on the face: the eyes, ears, nostrils, and mouth. These orifices play an important role in diagnosis in that the essential substances of the five *zàng* organs are understood as manifesting in particular orifices. Thus changes in the orifices are seen as reflective of pathological changes in the corresponding organs. *Qī* means "seven." *Qiào* means "orifice; a key to something."

> —*Any one of the openings of the body. The upper orifices or clear orifices are the eyes, ears, nostrils, and mouth, whereas the lower orifices or turbid orifices are the anal and genital orifices. These are collectively referred to as the nine orifices.*
>
> A PRACTICAL DICTIONARY OF CHINESE MEDICINE

> —*The condition of the five zàng can be read through the qī qiào.*
>
> LÍNG SHŪ, THE YELLOW EMPEROR'S CANON OF INTERNAL MEDICINE

Wǔ xīn

The five hearts—the palms, soles of the feet, and the chest. These five locations play an important role in diagnostic evaluation of particular conditions. The word *wǔ* means "five." The word *xīn* means "heart; the mind; feeling, intention; center."

Sì jí

The four extremities; the limbs. Also called *sì mò* or *sì wéi*. The term refers to the four limbs. The word *jí* means "limit, boundary, pole, border." The word *mò* means "tip, end; nonessential; final stage; powder, dust." The word *wéi* means "bind, hold together; maintain, preserve; thinking, thought, dimension."

> —*To get rid of accumulated fluids in the body, first one must gently shake the four extremities (sì mò).*
>
> SÙ WÈN, THE YELLOW EMPEROR'S CANON OF INTERNAL MEDICINE

> —*The four extremities are the basis of all yáng (in the body).*
>
> SÙ WÈN, THE YELLOW EMPEROR'S CANON OF INTERNAL MEDICINE

Words and Terms Related to Diagnosis and Etiology

Liù qì

1. The six excesses or untimeliness of the six *qì;* referring to wind, cold, damp, summerheat, dampness, dryness, and fire as pathogenic factors. This term is used to describe the environmental conditions which ancient theorists identified as pathogenic factors in etiology. When changes in weather exceed an individual's tolerance, disease results. Identifying which of the six *qì* are involved in the pathogenesis of a disease is an important step in diagnosis. 2. Six (types of) body substances; referring to essence, *qì,* liquid, humor, blood, and vessels (or pulse).

> —*Wind diseases are most common in spring, summerheat in summer, damp disease in long summer, dryness diseases in autumn, and cold diseases in winter. The Inner Canon (Nèi Jīng) referred to the six excesses as the "six qì" (the six kinds of weather), but recognized them as causes of diseases. Elementary Questions (Sù Wèn) states, "The hundred diseases are all engendered by wind, cold, summerheat, dampness, and fire."*
>
> A Practical Dictionary of Chinese Medicine
>
> —*The liù qì are the root of people's illness. Some arise internally. Some come from the external heavens.*
>
> Yī Biǎn

Qī qíng

The seven affects; referring to emotional as well as mental activities in general and their potential as pathogenic factors in the onset and progress of disease. Ancient theorists recognized that intense or prolonged emotional disturbance can act as a pathogenic factor and identified seven such states: anger, melancholy, anxiety, sorrow, terror, fright, and excessive joy. Each of these can act to disturb the normal function of the *qì,* blood, and viscera resulting in disease. This notion embraced thinking itself, which is understood as having the potential to exhaust the *qì* of the spleen if one thinks (or worries) excessively. The word *qī* means "seven." The word *qíng* means "feeling, affection, sentiment, emotion."

> —*Any natural movement of the heart, such as joy, anger, or grief. For example, The Book of Rites (Lǐ Jì) states, "What are the human affects? They are the seven things—joy, anger, grief, fear, love, loathing, and desire—of which a person is capable without learning."*

A PRACTICAL DICTIONARY OF CHINESE MEDICINE

Biàn zhèng

Pattern identification, referring to differential diagnosis in Chinese medicine, as in the phrase *biàn zhèng lùn zhì*, "identifying patterns and administering treatment." This term describes the clinical observation for making a diagnosis based on understanding the basic theories used to analyze and comprehend data as patterns of disease. The word *biàn* means "differentiate, distinguish, discriminate." The word *zhèng* means "prove, demonstrate; evidence; disease; symptom."

> —*A manifestation of human sickness indicating the nature, location, or cause of sickness. For example, the simultaneous presence of heat effusion, aversion to cold, and floating pulse forms an exterior pattern due to an external contraction; vigorous heat effusion, vexation and thirst, red tongue with yellow fur, and constipation constitutes an interior repletion pattern; wind stroke with clenched jaw, red face, rough breathing, phlegm-drool congestion, clenched hands, and a slippery stringlike or moderate sunken pulse constitutes a block pattern, whereas weak breathing, reversal cold in the limbs, pearly sweat, open mouth and closed eyes, open hands and enuresis, and faint fine pulse on the verge of expiration or sunken hidden pulse constitutes a desertion pattern. The concept of pattern is distinct from that of disease (as a specific kind of morbid condition).*

A PRACTICAL DICTIONARY OF CHINESE MEDICINE

WHO CAN RIDE THE DRAGON?

Bā gāng biàn zhèng

Eight-principle pattern identification, referring to differential diagnosis according to the eight fundamental principles. One of the basic methods of differential diagnosis which consists of determining the nature and location of pathological changes characterizing the patient's disease. This method includes an analysis of the conflict between the patient's resistance and the invading pathogenic influences. The eight principles, arranged in pairs, are: yīn and yáng; superficial and interior; cold and heat; and repletion and vacuity. Using this method, practitioners sort complex clinical manifestations into the appropriate categories in order to analyze and comprehend the patient's condition. The word *bā* means "eight." The word *gāng* means "key link; outline; program."

> —*Identification of disease patterns. Pattern identification is the process by which information gathered through four examinations (inspection, smelling and listening, inquiry, and palpation) is classified into different patterns. The first stage in the process is eight-principle pattern identification, in which four-examination data is classified as interior exterior, cold or heat, vacuity or repletion, and yīn and yáng. Depending on the results obtained, other pattern identification procedures are applied.*
>
> A PRACTICAL DICTIONARY OF CHINESE MEDICINE

Xū shí

Vacuity and repletion; also frequently translated as deficiency and excess, insubstantial and substantial (particularly in the martial arts), replete and deplete, full and empty. Referring to two principles for estimating the condition of both the patient's resistance and the pathogenic factors present. Vacuity generally refers to a general insufficiency of vitality, energy, and functioning of the body and is usually expressed in terms of yīn, yáng, *qì*, and blood. Repletion typically is used to refer to the hyperactivity of pathogenic factors and the resulting symptoms of conflict between the body's healthy resistance and these pathogenic factors. The word *xū* means "void, vacuous, emptiness, unoccupied; timid; weak; in poor health; insubstantial." The word *shí* means "solid; replete; true; real; reality; fact; substantial."

—Vacuity: emptiness or weakness. Repletion: fullness or strength. Vacuity is weakness of right qì, that is, the forces that maintain the health of the body and fight disease, whereas repletion is strength of evil qì or accumulation of physiological products within the body such as phlegm-rheum, water-damp, static blood, and stagnant qì. Vacuity patterns may be due to such causes as a weak constitution, damage to right qì either through enduring illness, loss of blood, seminal loss, and great sweating, or by invasion of an external evil (yáng evils readily damaging yīn humor and yīn evils readily damaging yáng qì). These causes are succinctly summed up in the phrase, "Where essential qì is despoliated, there is vacuity." Distinction is made between general insufficiencies of qì, blood, yīn, and yáng. Since these frequently affect specific organs, further distinction is made between such forms as heart yīn vacuity, liver blood vacuity, kidney yáng vacuity, and lung qì vacuity.

A PRACTICAL DICTIONARY OF CHINESE MEDICINE

Biǎo lǐ

External and internal; referring to two principal types of pattern identified according to the site and severity of the symptoms. Generally, diseases involving the skin, hair, and *jīng luò* are considered mild or superficial (*biǎo*). Those involving the viscera are considered more serious (*lǐ*), as they impair the interior. The word *biǎo* means "surface, outside, external." The word *lǐ* means "lining; inside, internal."

—Internal: "Located or arising within the body, especially of diseases due to excesses of the seven affects (internal damage) and evils resembling their external counterparts [e.g., internal wind, internal dampness].

External: Located or originating outside (the body), as in external evil.

A PRACTICAL DICTIONARY OF CHINESE MEDICINE

Hán rè

Cold and heat; referring to two of the eight-principle syndromes in differential diagnosis. These are considered to be the primary manifestations of yīn and yáng, i.e., symptoms that evidence a predominance of cold or heat. These two signs of disease are considered of primary importance in selection of herbal ingredients for prescriptions to treat illness. The word *hán* means "cold." The word *rè* means "heat."

—Cold: Cold in the body causing disease and classified as "cold" among the eight principles. The nature of cold as an evil and its clinical manifestations are similar to those of cold in the natural environment, e.g., low temperature, deceleration of activity, and congealing. Diseases caused by cold evil result from severe or sudden exposure to cold, e.g., catching cold, excessive consumption of cold fluids, or exposure to frost.

Heat: The opposite of cold. Heat is the manifestation of the sun and fire. Hot weather (and artificially heated environments) causes sweating, and without an adequate increase in fluid intake, thirst. There may be vexation and other discomforts naturally attributed to heat by the individual. In the healthy individual, these natural responses abate on exposure to cooler temperatures.

A PRACTICAL DICTIONARY OF CHINESE MEDICINE

Chuán biàn

Passage and transmutation, referring to the progress or development of disease, considered in various terms that tend to characterize the disease's progress and severity, thus establishing a basis for diagnosis as well as prognosis. The word *chuán* means "pass, pass on; hand down; transmit." The word *biàn* means "change; transmute; become; different; transform."

Zhèng xié

Righteous and evil; normal and pathogenic; referring to a distinction between the normal function of the organism as contrasted to the pathogenic changes accompanying and characterizing disease. These two words reflect a fundamental precept of Chinese medicine: that disease is a battle between the right *qì* and various pathogenic factors or evils that can originate both within and without the body proper. The word *zhèng* means "straight; right; righteous; main; honest; correct; principal; regular, normal; positive." The word *xié* means "evil; heretical; irregular."

> —*Right: Normal or rendering normal. Right complexion refers to the normal complexion of the healthy individual. Right* qì *denotes the forces that maintain normal bodily functions and that seek to re-establish them when evil* qì *is present. "Evil" stands in opposition to "right," the force that maintains health. Since evil actively fights right or summons activity of right to eliminate it, it is often called evil* qì. *Elementary Questions (Sù Wèn) states, "For evil to encroach, the* qì *must be vacuous."*
>
> A PRACTICAL DICTIONARY OF CHINESE MEDICINE

Wŭ yùn lìu qì

The five movements and six *qì*; the motion of the five phases and the six environmental phenomena. This ancient theory concerns the interrelationships that exist among the changes arising from the movement of the five phases (metal, water, wood, fire, and earth) and the six environmental phenomena (wind, cold, heat, damp, dry, and summerheat). These motions and their complex interrelationships are used to analyze and interpret the onset, development, proper treatment principle, and prognosis of disease. The word *yùn* means "motion; movement; carry; transport."

> —*The doctrine of five periods and six* qì *by which incidence of sickness is related to climate. The five periods are the five phases, i.e., wood, fire, earth, metal and water. The six* qì *are wind, heat, dampness, fire, dryness, and cold. The periods are calculated in terms of the ten heavenly stems, whereas the* qì *are calculated in terms of the twelve earthly branches. The doctrine aims, by means of the complementary opposition of* yīn *and* yáng *and the engendering and restraining relationship between the five phases, to calculate meteorological features and changes for each year and their effects on the human body.*
>
> A PRACTICAL DICTIONARY OF CHINESE MEDICINE

WHO CAN RIDE THE DRAGON?

—The changes of the qì in one's body obey the changes of the four seasons, the wŭ yùn and lìu qì. There is not one single instance where such changes disobey (this principle).

<small>Sù Wèn, The Yellow Emperor's Canon of Internal Medicine</small>

Sān bù jǐu hòu

Three positions and nine depths (for taking the pulse); referring to the three most common positions for feeling the pulse in the radial artery at the wrist joint, together with the three depths or levels of pressure applied by a doctor while palpating these three positions. In this definition, the three positions are known as *cùn, guān,* and *chǐ* and are located at the wrist joint on the radial aspect of the forearm, so that the pulse in the radial artery is felt beneath the fingertips. The three depths used to feel the pulse at each of these three positions (hence the nine depths) are used to determine various aspects of the condition of the pulse. The word *sān* means "three." The word *bù* means "part; section; unit; region; position." The word *jǐu* means "nine." The word *hòu* means "wait, await; inquire after; time; season; condition; state."

—An ancient pulse-taking scheme. In the context of the wrist pulse, the inch, bar, and cubit positions are the three positions, and the superficial level, mid-level, and deep level of each of these are the nine indicators.

<small>A Practical Dictionary of Chinese Medicine</small>

—Qi Bo said, "Man has three positions and three depths at each position. These are the places to diagnose all disease and make judgements concerning life and death [of the patient] to know how to adjust the insubstantial and substantial aspects of the constitution and thus eliminate illness." The Yellow Emperor inquired further, asking, "What are these three positions?" And Qi Bo answered, "The upper, the middle, and the lower positions [cùn, guān, chǐ]. Every position has three depths that represent heaven, earth, and mankind. One must use the finger tips to feel the pulse [at these positions] to ascertain the truth about the illness from sān bù jǐu hòu."

<small>Sù Wèn, The Yellow Emperor's Canon of Internal Medicine</small>

Cùn, guān, chǐ

The three positions for feeling the pulse located on the radial aspect of the forearm, near the wrist joint where the pulsation in the radial artery can be felt.

The styloid process of the radius serves as a landmark for locating the precise location of these positions, starting at the center, the *guān* position. The position just distal to the styloid process is *cùn*; the position proximal to the styloid process is *chǐ*. The word *cùn* is a unit of measure of length approximately equal to one inch. It also means "very little; small; short." The word *guān* means a "pass; juncture; to shut, close, turn off, lock up; concern; involve." The word *chǐ* is a unit of measure of length approximately equal to one foot or 1/3 of a meter. In ancient times it was determined, like the cubit, by the measure from the elbow to the wrist. Hence in Chinese medicine it often refers to the elbow or, as in this case, to sites located nearer to the elbow than others to which they are compared.

> —*The balance of qì, blood, yīn, and yáng manifests in the changes of cùn, the mouth of qì. Here one can determine the prognosis of an illness.*
>
> SÙ WÈN, THE YELLOW EMPEROR'S CANON OF INTERNAL MEDICINE

Jǔ àn xún

The three depths—releasing, pressing, and probing—employed in taking the pulse. These terms refer to the traditional method of palpating the pulse by varying the pressure applied to the fingertips. The lightest pressure is called *jǔ*, or "releasing." Moderate pressure is known as *àn*, or "pressing." Feeling for the deep part or the root of the pulse is done with heavier pressure known as *xún*, or "probing." While probing, the doctor will often shift the position of his or her fingers, searching for more information. The word *jǔ* means "lift; raise up; release; hold up." The word *àn* means "press; push down; restrain; control." The word *xún* means "look for; search; seek." It is also an ancient unit of measuring length equal to about eight *chǐ*.

WHO CAN RIDE THE DRAGON?

—There are three key points for pulse diagnosis: releasing, pressing, and probing.

Jǐng Yuè Quán Shū

Sì zhěn: *wàng zhěn, wén zhěn, wèn zhěn, qiè zhěn*

The four examinations. These are the four traditional methods of physical examination: *wàng zhěn*—visual inspection (looking at the patient); *wén zhěn*—listening (not only to what the patient says but to other sounds present in the patient's body) and smelling; *wèn zhěn*—inquiry, and *qiè zhěn*—palpation.

—The four examinations, inspection, listening and smelling, inquiry, and palpation, provide the raw data for diagnosis. Correlation of data from all four examinations is essential for complete diagnosis. The four examinations are followed by pattern identification.

A Practical Dictionary of Chinese Medicine

Wàng zhěn—Visual inspection; looking. The first and most fundamental method for gathering diagnostic information about the patient consists of looking at the patient's physical appearance, posture, mental and emotional status (as reflected in outward signs), color, and so forth. This includes inspection of urine, stool, and other secretions and excretions. For the well-trained doctor it includes a comprehensive inventory of all relevant data that can be gathered through observation. The word *wàng* means "inspection; looking with the eyes." The word *zhěn* means "pattern, diagnosis."

—One of the four examinations; looking at the patient and his phlegm, urine, and stool for diagnostic information. In inspection, attention is paid to the spirit, general physical appearance, and any part of the body where there is discomfort. Special attention focuses on the complexion and tongue, which are important indicators of the bowels and viscera.

A Practical Dictionary of Chinese Medicine

Wén zhěn—Listening and smelling. This diagnostic method consists of gathering data by means of the doctor's own olfactory and auditory organs. The doctor listens to the various sounds the patient makes—

such as voice, breathing, coughing, moaning—and notes any particular odors the patient emits. The word *wén* means "hear; smell."

> —*One of the four examinations; examination of the body by listening and smelling. In the Inner Canon (Nèi Jīng) the "listening and smelling" examination was limited to listening, and was primarily concerned with the the relationship of the five notes of the Chinese scale (gōng, shāng, jiǎo, zhǐ, and yǔ) and the five voices (shouting, laughing, singing, crying, and moaning) to the five viscera. In the Han Dynasty, Zhang Ji placed voice, breathing, panting, coughing, vomiting, and hiccough sounds within the listening and smelling examination. Since the Chinese wén means both listening and smelling, examination of smells was added to the scope of examination without any need for a change in name.*
>
> A PRACTICAL DICTIONARY OF CHINESE MEDICINE

Wèn zhěn—Inquiring, asking. This method consists of asking the patient for specific information concerning his or her present illness, history, dietary and other habits. In female patients it includes questions relative to menstruation and childbearing. Questions concern age, native region, occupation, and other aspects of the patient's daily activities. The word *wèn* means "ask, interrogate, examine."

> —*One of the four examinations; examination by questioning the patient or those attending him. According to Zhang Jing-Yue (Ming, 1563-1640), inquiry should be based on ten questions: 1. Heat effusion and aversion to cold. 2. Sweating. 3. Head and body. 4. Stool and urine. 5. Food and drink. 6. Chest. 7. Deafness. 8. Thirst. 9. Identifying yīn and yáng from the pulse and complexion. 10. Noting any odors or abnormalities of the spirit. The first eight of these items, actually the only ones that are essentially part of inquiry, are still to this day considered to apply.*
>
> A PRACTICAL DICTIONARY OF CHINESE MEDICINE

Qiè zhěn—Palpation. This method of physical examination consists of palpating various parts of the patient's body to investigate the condition of the pulse, the chest, the abdomen, and the extremities to help establish a diagnosis. The word *qiè* means "correspond to, be close to, be sure."

—One of the four examinations; the process of examining the surface of the body by touch to detect the presence of disease. The pulse examination, an essential part of routine examination, is the most common form of palpation. Palpation of other parts of the body is called body palpation.

A Practical Dictionary of Chinese Medicine

Shé zhĕn

Examination of the tongue; referring to the process of examining the tongue and its coating to determine its size, general appearance, relative moisture; thickness and color and characteristics of the coating. The word *shé* means "tongue."

—Inspection of the tongue and its fur (coating). The tongue examination provides some of the most important data for pattern identification. It can reveal the state of qì and blood, advance and regression of disease, the degree of heat and cold, and the depth of evil penetration. Changes in the appearance of the tongue are particularly pronounced in externally contracted heat (febrile) diseases and diseases of the stomach and spleen. However, in clinical practice, serious illnesses are not necessarily reflected in major changes in the appearance of the tongue. Furthermore, normal healthy individuals may show abnormal changes in the appearance of the tongue. Therefore, the data provided by the tongue examination must be carefully weighed against other signs, the pulse, and the patient's history, before an accurate diagnosis can be made.

A Practical Dictionary of Chinese Medicine

—The tongue manifests the condition of the heart. The coating shows clear signs of the condition of the stomach. By inspection of the tongue, one can predict the prosperity or decline of the righteous qì and understand the condition of the pathogenic qì.

Biàn Shé Zhí Nán

—If you identify the actual situation according to the constitution of the tongue, you won't make mistakes.

Lín Zhèng Yàn Shé Fă

Shí wèn

Ten questions; referring to the ten basic aspects of a patient that a doctor inquires about in gathering diagnostic information. These include feelings of heat or coldness; perspiration; condition of the head, trunk and limbs; urination and defecation; appetite; condition of the chest and abdomen; hearing and sleeping; thirst; (in female patients) menstruation, leukorrhea, and so forth, including the growth and nourishment of children; and past history and the cause of disease. The word *shí* means "ten." The word *wèn* means "question."

> —*When you enter a new country, you must ask about their customs. When you walk into others' homes, you must inquire as to their family affairs. When you walk into the court, rites. When a doctor begins to treat a patient, he must ask about all conditions.*
>
> LÍNG SHŪ, THE YELLOW EMPEROR'S CANON OF INTERNAL MEDICINE

Wŭ sè

The five colors; referring to the colors associated with the five phases and the five *zàng* organs. These are: green (a greenish-blue associated with wood, liver); red (fire, heart); yellow (earth, spleen); white (metal, lungs); and black (water, kidneys). Observation of these colors as they appear in the body is taken together with other clinical data and forms an important aspect of diagnosis. The word *sè* means color.

> —*Five colors manifest on the face. Here you can inspect the qì of the five zàng organs.*
>
> LÍNG SHŪ, THE YELLOW EMPEROR'S CANON OF INTERNAL MEDICINE
>
> —*If the five colors all appear at the same time, the disease is the result of a conflict of heat and cold.*
>
> SÙ WÈN, THE YELLOW EMPEROR'S CANON OF INTERNAL MEDICINE

Sān yīn

The three kinds of pathogenic factors; a method of classifying pathogenic factors in terms of their point of origin as endogenous, exogenous,

WHO CAN RIDE THE DRAGON?

or neutral (literally non-external–internal). These three categories are known as: *nèi yīn*, endogenous pathogenic factors which include abnormal emotional activities; *wài yīn*, exogenous pathogenic factors including wind, cold, summerheat, damp, dry, and fire; and *bù nèi wài yīn*, pathogenic factors which are neither endogenous nor exogenous, such as improper diet, fatigue, trauma, animal bites, insect stings, and fatigue. The word *yīn* means "cause, because of, as a result of." The word *nèi* means "inner, within, inside." The word *wài* means "outer, outward, outside, external."

> —*External, internal, and neutral causes of disease. The term "three causes" was coined by Chen Wu-Ze in his "A Unified Treatise on Diseases, Patterns, and Remedies According to the Three Causes (Sān Yīn Jí Yī Bìng Zhèng Fāng Lùn)" published in 1174 C.E. External factors are the six excesses. Internal causes are the seven affects. Neutral causes (literally "non-external-internal") include eating too much or too little, taxation fatigue, knocks and falls, crushing, drowning, and animal, insect, and reptile injuries.*
>
> A PRACTICAL DICTIONARY OF CHINESE MEDICINE

> —*A thousand sufferings fall into just three categories. First, the evil invades the jīng luò and enters the zàng fǔ. This is known as external causes. Second, blood and vessels connect the four limbs and nine orifices. When these become congested, illness follows. This is called internal causes. The third category contains such aspects as sexual life, wounds from knives, bites from insects and beasts. These are known as neither internal nor external."*
>
> JĪN GUÌ YÀO LÙE

Wèi qì yíng xuè biàn zhèng

Four-aspect pattern identification. Pattern identification by analysis of the *wèi, qì, yíng,* and *xuè* aspects or levels of the organism. This phrase refers to a diagnostic theory and method primarily used in determining the treatment of seasonal febrile diseases by estimating a location, nature, and prognosis. This theory provides four aspects or categories of disease, i.e., the *wèi* or external defensive layer, the *qì* or functional transformative layer, the *yíng* or nutritive layer, and the *xuè* or blood layer.

—According to doctrine of warm diseases, warm evils invade the body to first affect defense, and then progress, unless halted by right qì or treatment, through the other aspects. When disease affects defense, sweat-effusing treatment may be given. Only when it reaches the qì aspect can qì-clearing treatment be prescribed. When it enters construction, treatment involves outthrusting heat to the qì aspect. Finally, when it reaches blood and causes depletion and frenetic movement, blood cooling and dissipation is prescribed.

A PRACTICAL DICTIONARY OF CHINESE MEDICINE

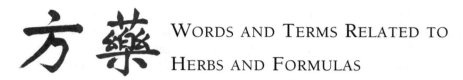

WORDS AND TERMS RELATED TO HERBS AND FORMULAS

According to legend, Shen Nong, one of the prehistoric "emperors" (along with the Yellow Emperor and Fu Xi), tasted hundreds of plants in his quest to find those with healing properties. Shen Nong was the first to develop an understanding that individual plants—and even various parts of the same plant—have different natures, flavors, and functions. This understanding led to the organizational classifications of the Chinese herbal materia medica.

Sì qì sì xìng

1. The four natures of medicinals; 2. the four qì of medicinals; 3. temperature (when applied to medicinals). This term refers to the essential nature of medicinal herbs with respect to their therapeutic effects and synergistic characteristics. These four natures are: cold, hot, cool, and warm. They are categorized according to yīn and yáng. Hot and warm are in the yáng category; cold and cool are in the yīn category.

The purpose of categorizing medicinal substances in this fashion is to permit herbal practitioners to follow a basic precept of Chinese herbal medicine: "use heat to overcome cold pathogenic factors; use cold to overcome hot pathogenic factors." Herbs with a cold nature are typically used to clear hot or warm pathogenic factors as well as internally generated heat. They are used in treating heat patterns and yáng patterns. Herbs with a hot nature are usually used to dispel cold pathogenic factors by warming the interior, invigorating yáng, and nourishing qì. They are used in treatment of cold patterns and yīn patterns. The word *xìn* means "nature."

> *—The four natures of medicinals, cold, heat, warmth, and coolness. Cold medicinals are ones effective in treating heat patterns, whereas hot medicinals are those effective in treating cold patterns. Warm and cool medicinals are medicinals with mild hot or cold natures. In addition, there is also a balanced nature whose nature is neither predominantly hot nor cold.*
>
> A PRACTICAL DICTIONARY OF CHINESE MEDICINE

Wŭ wèi

The five flavors; referring to the tastes of herbs: acrid, sweet, sour, bitter, and salty. These flavors are understood to correspond with the five *zàng* organs according to the following arrangement: heart–bitter; liver–sour; spleen–sweet; lungs–acrid; and kidney–salty. The word *wèi* means "flavor."

> *—According to Elementary Questions (Sù Wèn), the flavors can be classified as yīn and yáng: "Acrid and sweet effusing (i.e., diaphoretic) and dissipating medicinals are yáng; sour and bitter upwelling (i.e., emetic) and discharging (i.e., draining) medicinals are yīn; salty upwelling and discharging medicinals are yīn; bland percolating and discharging medicinals are yáng." According to the Comprehensive Herbal Foundation (Běn Cǎo Gāng Mù) there is a relationship between flavor and bearing: "no sour or salty medicinals bear upward; no sweet or acrid ones bear downward. No cold medicinals float; no hot ones sink."*
>
> A PRACTICAL DICTIONARY OF CHINESE MEDICINE

> *—Each of the five flavors will enter the organ which favors it.*
>
> LÍNG SHŪ, THE YELLOW EMPEROR'S CANON OF INTERNAL MEDICINE

> *—The five flavors of herbs enter the five zàng organs. Either supplement or drain according to the nature of the herbs employed.*
>
> BĚN CǍO GĀNG MÙ

Guī jīng

Channel entry; referring to the theory that different medicinals enter and affect different channels and their related organs. This theory is based on the theory of the *zàng fǔ* (q.v.), the theory of *jīng luò* (q.v.), and the nature and flavor of the various medicinals. For example, *Radix Platycodi*, an herb with an acrid flavor, is effective for treating cough due to impairment of the function of the lung. This herb is said to enter the lung channel. Herbs that distribute their effect to two or more channels have more widespread effects on the organism and are therefore more useful in treatment.

This theory of correspondence or distribution to the various channels appears in the *Yellow Emperor's Canon of Internal Medicine*: "The sour enters the liver. The acrid enters the lung. The bitter enters the heart. The salty enters the kidney. The sweet enters the spleen. This is called the five entrances." The word *guī* means "to go back to, return; give back to, return something to someone; converge, come together; turn over to; put into someone's charge."

> —*Action (of a medicinal) on a particular channel and the organ to which the channel homes. For example, platycodon (jié gěng) and tussilago (kuǎn dōng huā) treat cough and panting and are said to enter the lung channel; gastrodia (tiān má), scorpion, (quán xiē) and antelope horn (líng yáng jiǎo) treat convulsions and are said to enter the liver channel.*
>
> A PRACTICAL DICTIONARY OF CHINESE MEDICINE

Jūn chén zuǒ shǐ

Medicinal roles—sovereign, minister, assistant, and courier. The designations given to medicinal ingredients based upon the role they play within a prescription.

The words are taken from the nomenclature of the imperial court and function metaphorically to identify the relative importance and functions of the key herbs in an herbal prescription. The word *jūn* means "sovereign or monarch." It is sometimes translated as "king." In herbal formulas it refers to the chief herb in the formula, that is, the main active medicinal. The word *chén* means "minister." The *chén* ingredient in a formula serves to intensify the action of the *jūn*. The word *zuǒ* means "assistant or adjuvant." In herbal formulas, the *zuǒ* ingredient can play different roles, for example, reducing the secondary effects or toxicity of the *jūn* medicinal. The word *shǐ* means "courier or guide." The *shǐ* herb in a formula has the function of directing the effect of the formula to the target organ or channel. It can also serve to balance the entire formula. *Shǐ* also means "send, tell somebody to do something; use, apply; envoy; messenger; cause, make."

> —*The sovereign performs the principal action of the formula, addressing the principal sign pattern. The sovereign may be one or more medicinals. The minister provides direct assistance to the sovereign. The assistant addresses secondary patterns or reduces the toxicity or harshness of the sovereign. The courier makes other medicinals act on the desired part of the body or harmonizes the other medicinals.*
>
> A PRACTICAL DICTIONARY OF CHINESE MEDICINE

> —*The herbs in a formula have the positions of sovereign, minister, assistant, and courier, to promote, control, and harmonize with one another.*
>
> SHÉN NÓNG BĚN CǍO JĪNG

 # CATEGORIES FOR CLASSIFYING HERBS

Herbs are traditionally categorized according to their primary function. There are eighteen such categories comprising the standard herbal materia medica.

Jiě biǎo

Exterior resolution; this refers to herbs that have the ability to expel external (superficial) pathogenic factors. The word *jiě* means "resolve; separate, divide; undo; alloy; dispel; dismiss; solve." The word *biǎo* means "surface."

*—The method of resolving the exterior takes various forms depend-
ing on the evil. See the entries listed below.*

*Resolving the exterior with coolness and acridity (qīng liáng jiě
biǎo)*

*Resolving the exterior with warmth and acridity (qīng wēn jiě
biǎo)*

Enrich yīn and resolve the exterior (zī yīn jiě biǎo)

Boosting qì and resolving the exterior (bǔ qì jiě biǎo)

Assisting yáng and resolving the exterior (zhù yáng jiě biǎo)

Resolving the flesh (jiě jī)

Outthrusting papules (tòu zhěn)

Coursing the exterior (shū biǎo)

A PRACTICAL DICTIONARY OF CHINESE MEDICINE

Qīng rè

Clearing heat; this refers to medicinals that have the ability to dispel or
clear heat. The word *qīng* means "clear." The word *rè* means "heat."

*—Clearing heat is used in the treatment of interior heat patterns
such as qì-aspect heat, blood-aspect heat, damp-heat, and yáng
sore patterns. Clearing heat is a generic term that corresponds to
clearing among the eight methods. It includes clearing heat (in a
more specific sense), draining fire, and resolving toxin.*

A PRACTICAL DICTIONARY OF CHINESE MEDICINE

Xiè xià

Draining precipitation. The word *xiè* means "drain, discharge, rush
down; pour out; have loose bowels." The word *xià* "means down, lower,
inferior, below, downward."

*A method of treatment used to eliminate fire from the heart region,
i.e., from the stomach or the heart itself. This method applies to
both a) exuberant stomach fire with sore swollen gums, bad breath,*

WHO CAN RIDE THE DRAGON?

clamoring stomach, constipation, red tongue with yellow fur, and a rapid pulse; and b) exuberant heart fire with frenetic movement of the blood (blood ejection, spontaneous external bleeding), constipation, reddish urine, red eye, mouth sores, yellow tongue fur, and rapid pulse.

A PRACTICAL DICTIONARY OF CHINESE MEDICINE

Xiāo dǎo

Abductive dispersion. Medicinals in this category are used to strengthen the spleen and regulate the *qì*. They are often used in formulas for treatment of indigestion, flatulence, and syndromes in which such symptoms are prominent or present. The word *xiāo* means "disappear, vanish; dispel; remove." The word *dǎo* means "lead, guide; transmit, conduct."

—*Dispersing food and abducting stagnation, often called abductive dispersion, is employed in the treatment of food stagnation causing oppression in the stomach duct and abdominal distention, poor appetite, putrid belching, swallowing of upflowing acid, and nausea and upflow, abdominal pain, constipation, or diarrhea with ungratifying defecation.*

A PRACTICAL DICTIONARY OF CHINESE MEDICINE

Huà tán zhǐ ké píng chuǎn

Transforming phlegm, suppressing cough, and calming asthma. The word *huà* means "change, transform; dissolve; burn up." The word *tán* means "phlegm." The word *zhǐ* means "stop." The word *kè* means "cough." The word *píng* means "flat, smooth, calm, peaceful, quiet; put down, suppress." The word *chuǎn* means "breathe heavily, gasp for breath; asthma."

—*Any method of treatment used to eliminate phlegm gently. The method of transforming phlegm takes different forms depending on the location and cause of the phlegm pattern.*

A PRACTICAL DICTIONARY OF CHINESE MEDICINE

Lì qì

Disinhibiting *qì*. Medicinals in this category are used to restore the patency of the *qì*. They have the effect of making *qì* that has stopped moving and transforming once again resume its normal interactions. The word *lì* "means advantage, benefit, profit; favorable; sharp."

> —*To promote fluency, movement, or activity, i.e., to treat inhibited flow of qì, blood, or fluids, or inhibited physical movement.*
> A PRACTICAL DICTIONARY OF CHINESE MEDICINE

Lì xuè

Disinhibiting blood. Herbs in this category are used to nourish, enrich, cool, or warm the blood. They can be used to eliminate blood stasis and promote blood circulation as well as to stop bleeding.

Qū fēng shèng shī

Dispelling wind and overcoming dampness. Herbs in this category are used to treat invasion and accumulation of wind and dampness. The word *qū* means "dispel; remove; drive away." The word *fēng* means "wind." The word *shèng* means "victory, success; surpass, be superior to." The word *shī* means "wet, damp, humid."

> —*A method of treatment used to address wind-damp lodged in the channels and network vessels, the flesh, and the joints that causes wandering pain . . .*
> A PRACTICAL DICTIONARY OF CHINESE MEDICINE

Lì niào shèn shī

Disinhibiting urination to overcome dampness. Herbs in this category are used as diuretics in treatment of patterns characterized by accumulation of dampness due to hypoactivity of the urinary system. The word *niào* means "urine." The word *shèn* means "ooze; seep."

WHO CAN RIDE THE DRAGON?

Wēn lǐ

Warming the interior. Herbs in this category are used in the treatment of syndromes characterized by accumulation of cold in the interior of the body. The word *wēn* means "warm; warm up." The word *lǐ* means "inner; inside."

Fāng xiāng huà shī

Transforming turbidity with aroma. Herbs in this category are aromatic, fragrant herbs used to transform dampness and restore consciousness. The word *fāng* means "sweet-smelling, fragrant." The word *xiāng* means "aromatic, fragrant, scented." The word *huà* means "transform, change, dissolve."

> —*Transforming turbidity with aroma is used to treat distention and oppression in the abdomen and stomach duct, accompanied by upflow nausea and desire to vomit, thin sloppy stool, fatigue and lack of strength, and a slimy sensation and sweet taste in the mouth.*
>
> A PRACTICAL DICTIONARY OF CHINESE MEDICINE

Fāng xiāng kāi qiào

Opening the orifices with fragrant herbs. These herbs are specifically used to open the orifices of *qì* and *shén* and thus restore consciousness when it has lapsed. The word *kāi* means "to open." The word *qiào* means "orifice, aperture, opening; a key to something."

> —*A method of treatment used to address clouded spirit and coma due to evil obstructing the orifices of the heart. Opening the orifices employs acrid aromatic penetrating medicinals which penetrate the heart and free the orifices, repel foulness, and open blocks. Opening the orifices is applied in the treatment of sudden clouding reversal (clouding of consciousness due to abnormal qì flow) in diseases such as fright wind, epilepsy, wind stroke, or angina pectoris, or in coma caused by internal block occurring in externally contracted heat (febrile) disease.*
>
> A PRACTICAL DICTIONARY OF CHINESE MEDICINE

Bŭ yì

Supplement and boost. Herbs in this category are generally used to build and nourish the body. The category itself is typically discussed in four subcategories: herbs that invigorate the *qì*; herbs that nourish the blood; herbs that engender *yīn*; and herbs that invigorate *yáng*. The word *bŭ* means "mend, patch, repair; fill; supply; make up for; nourish; benefit; help." The word *yì* means "benefit, profit, advantage, increase."

> —*To increase or strengthen. Yīn, yáng, qì, and blood may all be supplemented; the organs that most commonly receive supplementation are the spleen and kidney. Because supplementation is often associated with qì, the term is frequently seen together with the word boost.*
>
> A Practical Dictionary of Chinese Medicine

Gù sè

Astriction to secure. Herbs in this category are used to treat patterns characterized by loss of essence, *qì*, blood, or body fluids. The word *gù* means "solid, firm, firmly; fluid." The word *sè* means "puckered, astringent; not smooth; hard-going."

> —*Securing and astriction involves the use of supplementing and astringent medicinals to constrain sweat in the treatment of spontaneous or night sweating; constrain the lung in the treatment of persistent cough; astringe the intestines in the treatment of persistent diarrhea culminating in prolapse of the anus (termed "enduring diarrhea efflux desertion"); secure essence in the treatment of seminal emission or seminal efflux; reduce urine in the treatment of copious urine or enuresis; stanch bleeding to treat severe bleeding; secure the menses to treat flooding and spotting; or check vaginal discharge to treat persistent vaginal discharge.*
>
> A Practical Dictionary of Chinese Medicine

Ān shén

Quieting the spirit. These medicinals are used to calm the mind and sedate the body. The word *ān* means "calm; peaceful." The word *shén* means "spirit; god; supernatural, magical; mind."

—A method of treatment used to address disquieted spirit (heart palpitations, insomnia, agitation, mania).

A PRACTICAL DICTIONARY OF CHINESE MEDICINE

Píng gān xī fēng

Calming the liver to extinguish internal wind. Medicinals in this category are sedative in nature and are used to treat patterns characterized by hyperactivity of the liver resulting in internal wind, the typical pattern being wind stroke or apoplexy. The word *píng* means "quieted down, peaceful, calm." The word *gān* means "liver." The word *xī* means "extinguish, stop, cease, rest." The word *fēng* means "wind."

—A method of treatment used to address ascendant liver yáng stirring internal wind with pulling pain in the head, dizziness, deviated eyes and mouth, numbness or tremor of the limbs, stiffening of the tongue, deviated trembling tongue, unclear speech, red tongue with thin fur, a stringlike pulse, and, in severe cases, clouding collapse, hypertonicity or convulsions of the limbs.

A PRACTICAL DICTIONARY OF CHINESE MEDICINE

Qū chóng

Expelling worms and parasites. These are anti-helminthic herbs. The word *qū* means to "drive out, expel, disperse." The word *chóng* means "worm."

Wài yòng

External use. The word *wài* means "outside, external." The word *yòng* means "use, usefulness."

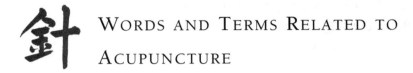

針 WORDS AND TERMS RELATED TO ACUPUNCTURE

Acupuncture is a specialization of Chinese medicine. It relies on much of the basic theory of the subject and includes its own extensive body of theories, concepts, and terms.

Zhēn jiǔ

Literally, this term translates as "needle" and "long-lasting fire." Together, these two words form the term that is typically translated into English as "acupuncture and moxibustion" or "acumoxa therapy," and commonly referred to simply as "acupuncture." It refers to two allied forms of therapy, *zhēn fǎ* and *jiǔ fǎ*. *Zhēn fǎ* refers to the therapeutic method of applying any of a variety of types of needles, including filiform needles, three-edged needles, plum-blossom needles, and intradermal needles, among others.

The application of such needles is conducted to stimulate certain points that lie along channels for the treatment of disease. *Jiǔ fǎ* consists of the application of an herb, artemisia, which is prepared in various ways and then burned either near or on certain points to warm and thereby stimulate the movement of *qì*.

The meaning of the word *jiǔ* is of interest. It is composed of two other characters. The one on top is also pronounced *jiǔ* and means "long, long-lasting, long ago." The bottom character is *huǒ*, "fire." These two, taken as a unit, can be understood to mean "long-lasting fire," and indeed this is a clear reflection of the therapeutic principle of moxibustion—to stimulate the movement of *qì* by warming certain points for a period of time. Such stimulation at particular points is also understood to increase heat in related organs, remote regions of the body, and the body as a whole. *Fǎ* is a word with numerous related meanings, including "law," "method," "way," "follow," "model," "standard," and "magic arts," among others.

Shū xué

Transport point; this is a term for a category of acupoints found on the back in two lines, one approximately one and one-half inches lateral to the spine and the other at about three inches lateral to the spine. These points are related to the functioning of the internal organs and various other aspects of physiology. The word *shū* means "transport; communication." The word *xué* means "acupuncture point." (See Chapter 1 for a complete definition of *xué*.)

Mù xué

Alarm points; referring to a group of points on the anterior surface of the body which have both diagnostic and therapeutic interrelationships with the internal organs. The *qì* of the various organs is understood to gather and collect at corresponding *mù xué* as a result and thus signal pathological changes. As these changes in the *qì* frequently precede any other clinical symptoms or signs, the *mù xué* points can "sound an alarm" prior to the onset of disease. The word *mù* means to "collect, gather, or muster together." It is used in phrases referring to the gathering together of troops or the collection of taxes. Thus the sense of "alarm" as the term is usually translated into English arises from the military metaphor.

Wǔ shū xué

Five transport points; referring to a group of points on each of the twelve primary channels including: well points; spring points; stream points; river points; and uniting (sea) points. Here the word *shū* means transportation or communication. It features importantly in the nomenclature of acupuncture points in general and is an important clue to the nature of the *jīng luò* system as a physiological information transmission and storage system. In this usage it underscores a metaphoric image of the *qì* likened to water as it moves from its sources in the extremities towards its pooling places on its journey towards the torso and the viscera. The well points are the most distal on each channel. The metaphor continues through spring, stream, river, and sea as the *qì* travels through the channels towards the interior of the body.

Yíng suí bǔ xiè

Directional supplementation and drainage; referring to two basic methods of insertion and stimulation of acupuncture needles when they are inserted in the patient. Supplementation has often been called "tonification" in English. It is typically accomplished by inserting the needle so that its tip is angled in the same direction as the *qì* moves through the channel on which the point chosen for insertion lies. This method includes slight movement of the needle once it has been inserted. Draining is typically accomplished so that the tip of the needle is angled in the opposite direction as the *qì* moves. This action is followed by more intense stimulation of the needle. The word *yíng* means "to go to meet; greet; receive; move towards." The word *suí* means "follow; comply with; adapt to; let, allow; along with." The word *bǔ* means "supplement, mend, patch, repair; fill, supply; nourish; benefit; reinforce." The word *xiè* means "flow swiftly; rush down; pour out; drain; to have loose bowels; to have diarrhea."

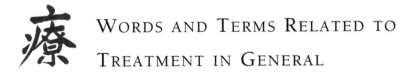

WORDS AND TERMS RELATED TO TREATMENT IN GENERAL

Herbal medicine and acupuncture are two of the many aspects of Chinese medicine. Though it is beyond the scope of this book to delve into other areas of specialization, we present here several terms that convey the theories, concepts, and principles of treatment in general.

Bā fǎ

Eight methods (of medical treatment); referring to the eight basic therapeutic principles.

> —A classification of medicinal treatment methods by Cheng Zhong-Ling of the Qing Dynasty under the eight rubrics: sweating, ejection, precipitation, harmonization, warming, clearing, supplementation, and dispersion.
>
> A PRACTICAL DICTIONARY OF CHINESE MEDICINE

Yīn píng yáng mì

A state when yīn is calm and yáng is sound. Yīn and yáng in equilibrium; referring to the ideal state in which yīn and yáng are interregulated and remain in harmonious balance, continually adjusting so as to maintain the homeostasis of the entire organism. This results in a healthy body and mind. This is the conceptual equivalent of homeostasis in the sense that it is understood in Western physiology. The word píng means "calm, flat, on the same level, even, smooth, equal, average, common, ordinary." The word mì means "close, dense, thick, intimate, meticulous, sound."

> —When yīn and yáng are in harmony the jīng and shén are well regulated. If yīn and yáng are separated the jīng qì will be exhausted.
>
> SÙ WÈN, THE YELLOW EMPEROR'S CANON OF INTERNAL MEDICINE

Yīn rén zhì yí

"Act according to person. Treat disease according to individual patients: different patient, different treatment." This phrase refers to a fundamental concept in Chinese medicine, which is that disease manifests differently in different individuals. Therefore effective treatment must be tailored to each individual. This takes into account differences not only in the manifestations of disease but in each patient's constitution and disease history. The word yīn means "reason, cause; according to." The word *rén* means "person, people." The word *zhì* means "make; work out; formulate; restrict; control; system." The word *yí* means "suitable, appropriate, fitting." The phrase literally says, "Work out [treatment] suitable to fit the person." It is the principle behind such statements as the following from the *Sù Wèn:*

> —*Give strong herbs to people who can take them. Use mild herbs for people who cannot take strong herbs.*
>
> Sù Wèn, The Yellow Emperor's Canon of Internal Medicine

Yīn dì zhì yí

"Act according to place. Treat diseases differently in different places; treatment should be fit to the environment." This phrase, like the one above, expresses a fundamental precept of treatment in Chinese medicine. Diseases manifests differently in different environments. For instance, a damp, hot environment will give rise to different symptoms and diseases than a cold, dry one. The human body interacts with the environment in subtle and profound ways; thus medical treatment must accord with the particular conditions of any given environment. The word *dì* means "earth; place; location, area." Literally, the phrase means, "Work out [treatment] suitable to the place [in which the treatment is given]."

> —*The Yellow Emperor asked, "Why are there many ways to treat disease?" Qi Bo answered, "This is due to the physical features of a place."*
>
> Sù Wèn, The Yellow Emperor's Canon of Internal Medicine

Yīn shí zhì yí

"Act according to time. Treat diseases differently at different times." This phrase expresses the third aspect of the principle of tailoring medical treatment to the individual, their environment, and the specific time. The word *shí* means "time; season." Literally, the phrase means, "Work out [treatment] suitable to the season [time] at which the treatment is given."

—Herbs with cold natures cannot be used in cold weather. Herbs with cool natures cannot be used in cool weather. Herbs with warm natures cannot be used in warm weather. Herbs with hot natures cannot be used in hot weather. This principle should be followed with respect to diet as well.

SÙ WÈN, THE YELLOW EMPEROR'S CANON OF INTERNAL MEDICINE

Tóng bìng yì zhì

"Unlike treatment of like disease. Same disease, different treatment." This phrase refers to another basic precept of Chinese medicine. Variations in the ways in which one disease manifests require that diseases be treated differently based on individual circumstances. This phrase sums up this notion that the same disease can require different treatments. The word *tóng* means "same." The word *yì* means "different, other, another."

—Qi Bo said, "The method of treating the qì in the Northwest regions should be to disperse and cool, for the cold weather favors a diet of hot food. Thus internal heat results. The method of treating the qì in the Southeast regions should be to gather and warm, because the hot weather favors a diet of cold food. Thus internal cold results. This is what is known as treating the same disease with different methods."

SÙ WÈN, THE YELLOW EMPEROR'S CANON OF INTERNAL MEDICINE

Tuī ná

Massage; a general name for massage or massotherapy. The word *tuī* means "push, push forward, promote." The word *ná* means to "hold, to take, to grasp." *Tuī ná* thus means pushing and holding, i.e., massage.

—The dào of tuī ná was called àn mó in ancient times. This is the method the ancients used to treat the body with their fingers instead of needles.

MÌ CHUÁN TUĪ NÁ MIÀO JUÉ

Key Terms of Chinese Medicine

Àn mó

Massage; another general term for massage and massotherapy. The word *àn* means "press, push down, keep one's hand on (something)." The word *mó* means "to rub, scrape, touch." *Àn mó* is a method of preventing and treating diseases using various massage techniques and methods as well as undertaking manipulation and adjustment of the joints and of the extremities. More specifically, *àn mó* is one of the eight manipulations used in bone setting in order to relax muscle tissue, dissipate blood stasis, and reduce swelling.

> —*Thus àn mó is for opening blockages and diverting yīn and yáng.*
> WANG BING'S COMMENTARY ON THE *SÙ WÈN*

 HEALTH PRESERVATION AND EXERCISE

An important part of Chinese medicine is the discipline of preserving health and extending life. Foremost among the various methods that fall in this category are exercises and disciplines aimed at cultivating the inborn treasures of the body, mind, and spirit. These are briefly described below.

Qì gōng

Qì or breathing exercise; referring to a variety of traditional practices consisting of physical, mental, and spiritual exercises. The regulation of the breath (*qì*) is a common feature of such exercise methods. The word *gōng* means "achievement, result; skill; work; exercise." It is composed of two radicals. The radical on the left is also pronounced *gōng* and means work. The radical on the right is the word *lì* and means strength or force. *Qì gōng* can be understood as exercise designed to strengthen and harmonize the *qì*, regulate the body and mind, and calm the spirit.

Tài jí quán

Grand ultimate boxing; also known as yīn-yáng boxing. *Tài jí quán* probably originated in the Song Dynasty as a method of physical, mental, and spiritual cultivation. It was first practiced by Daoist monks as a refinement of older *dǎo yǐn* exercises (see below). Both are methods used to incorporate philosophical precepts into daily life. *Tài jí quán* is a martial as well as a meditative art. Thus it has complementary aspects that combine in a comprehensive discipline of physical culture and mental and spiritual discipline. The word *quán* means "fist; boxing; punch."

Dǎo yǐn

Meditation and breathing exercises that seek to develop the ability to lead and guide the *qì* throughout the body for the benefit of the spirit, mind, and body. *Dǎo yǐn* exercises have a long history in China. They consist of bending, stretching, and otherwise mobilizing the extremities and the joints in order to free the flow of *qì* throughout the whole body. Like *qì gōng, dǎo yǐn* emphasizes control of the breath (*qì*). *Dǎo yǐn* also includes self-massage techniques which when practiced in combination with the other techniques serve to relieve fatigue and prolong life by activating and harmonizing the circulation of blood and *qì*. These techniques also stress the development of strength in the muscles and bones. The word *dǎo* means "lead, guide; transmit, conduct; instruct." The word *yǐn* means "draw; stretch; lead, guide; keep clear of; make way for; lure."

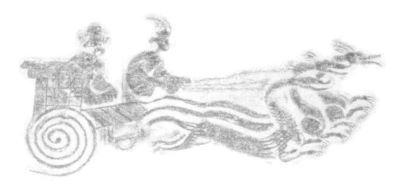

Before Completion

As scientific understanding has grown, so has our world become dehumanized. Man feels himself isolated in the cosmos, because he is no longer involved in nature and has lost his emotional "unconscious identity" with natural phenomena. These have slowly lost their symbolic implications. Thunder is no longer the voice of an angry god, nor is lightning his avenging missile. No river contains a spirit, no tree is the life principle of a man, no snake the embodiment of wisdom, no mountain cave the home of a great demon. No voices now speak to man from stones, plants, and animals, nor does he speak to them believing they can hear. His contact with nature has gone, and with it has gone the profound emotional energy that this symbolic connection supplied.

—CARL JUNG

PERHAPS ONE OF THE MORE USEFUL WAYS to account for the recent popularity of Chinese medicine is that it holds out a powerful and attractive hope to modern people who have lived for decades in a world so eloquently described by Carl Jung in the passage above. How can mankind survive without this profound emotional energy? Disconnected from the natural world, what becomes of us? Today, both the rapid growth of scientific knowledge, and the resultant expansion of technological frontiers threaten to drive humanity deeper and deeper into the "dehumanized" state about which Jung admonished us in 1964.

Yet recent trends in public demand for the so-called "alternative" forms of healing suggest that humanity is still very much in possession of the urge to stay connected with the natural world. In 1995, Harvard Medical School published a report that included statistical evidence that seven out of ten patients in the United States have tried some form of complementary medicine. This is a huge proportion.

Indeed, it is the patient population that is leading the way in this revolution of medical and healthcare delivery. But why are so many patients turning to alternative and complementary forms of medicine? It is easy to understand why doctors and medical clinics, HMOs, and medical schools are beginning to embrace complementary forms of medicine—not only to simplify and to lower costs, but to keep the trust and patronage of numerous patients who have found benefit in these forms of treatment. Yet what are these patients searching for? What are they finding?

No doubt there are many answers to why people decide to see an acupuncturist, homeopath, herbalist, or other non-conventional practitioner. Although we have no formal scientific evidence to justify our opinion, we strongly suspect that a common motivation is a desire for better communication. When people suffer they want to be heard and understood. Of course, they want to be healed and relieved of their suffering, but the satisfaction of the desire for communication is very probably an essential step in the healing process.

Chinese medicine has this to offer. The "split" between man and nature, which Jung and many others in the West have tried to understand and to "heal" for many years now, has never touched traditional Chinese philosophy. The impetus driving the development of Western sciences, technologies, and medicine—the urge to "conquer" nature—never drove China's ancient philosophers. Chinese thinkers and particularly Chinese doctors have, since ancient times, sought to live in harmony with nature. The classical Cartesian dichotomy which has paradoxically benefited and plagued the development of modern Western civilization simply cannot be found in the theoretical materials of Chinese medicine.

We propose that medicine, and particularly Chinese medicine, is best understood in the framework of its culture. Indeed, healing itself is a process rooted in a series of doctor–patient interactions that depend on an exchange of information and ideas mediated by cultural values. Among these cultural values, none is more basic than language. Thus we offer this work as a contribution to the healing process itself.

Select Annotated Bibliography

BOOKS IN ENGLISH

Cheng Man Qing, translated by Tam Gibbs, *Lao Tzu, My Words Are Very Easy to Understand,* Berkeley: North Atlantic Books, 1983

> This is one of the best English language versions of the Daoist classic of Lao Zi. It consists of the Chinese text followed by Professor Cheng's lecture notes on each chapter. The lectures took place at Professor Cheng's School of Correct Timing in New York in the early 1970's prior to Cheng's departure from New York and subsequent death in Taiwan. It is a bilingual edition which makes it particularly useful to serious students.

Fenellosa, Ernest, *The Chinese Written Character as A Medium for Poetry,* San Francisco: City Lights, 1963

> A seminal work on the understanding and appreciation of Chinese characters by non-Chinese, this lengthy essay was edited into its published form by Ezra Pound. Fenellosa's point of view continues to spark controversy among sinologists and linguists, but beyond the fine points of academic debate, the text is an indispensable introduction to the nature of the ancient Chinese language.

Fromkin, Victoria and Rodman, Robert, *An Introduction to Language,* New York: Harcourt Brace, 1993

> A primer on linguistics and theories of language, this book provides an overview of widely held theories and beliefs about language. It is highly readable, informative and instructive for those who wish to enter the world of linguistics.

Henricks, Robert G., *Lao-Tzu Te-Tao Ching, A New Translation Based on the Recently Discovered Ma-wang-tui Texts,* New York: Ballantine Books, 1989

> This book provides those who wish to engage in textual comparison and analysis with a valuable tool for penetrating beneath the surface in understanding the basic Daoist classic.

Lau, D.C. *Tao Te Ching,* New York: Penguin Books, 1963

> D.C. Lau's translation of Lao Zi is one of the oldest and best available. To a great extent it has served as a standard for subsequent English language versions of the text.

Lin Yu Tang, *My Country, My People,* New York: Reynal & Hitchcock, 1935

> Lin Yu Tang was one of China's leading intellectuals in the period between the end of the Qing dynasty and the establishment of the People's Republic. This book provides English language readers with something that is extremely rare: an insightful, loving, and frank assessment of China and her people as only a native son can offer, written in extraordinarily lucid English prose. An indispensable book for anyone who seeks to understand the Chinese people.

Lo, Benjamin *et al., Essence of Tai Chi Chuan, The Literary Tradition,* Berkeley: North Atlantic Books, 1981

> This is one of the first English-language translations of the classic texts of *tài jí quán.* It is also the best. The translators bring their considerable skill and experience in *tài jí quán* to the task of rendering extremely difficult Chinese text into meaningful English. Their work provides students of *tài jí quán* and Chinese philosophy and culture with rare insights.

Needham, Joseph *et al., Science and Civilization in China,* London: Oxford University Press. 1952 *passim*

> The seminal work on Chinese science, this series of books establishes a strong foundation for investigation of the contributions that the Chinese people have made to human knowledge and understanding of the world over 2000 years.

Needham, Joseph, *Science in Traditional China,* Cambridge: Harvard University Press, 1982

> In 1981, Needham gave a series of lectures at the Chinese University of Hong Kong. This book contains these lectures, which give readers an opportunity to hear the lucid considerations of one of the world's leading sinologists.

Pound, Ezra (tr.), *Confucius,* New York: New Directions, 1972

Pound was one of the most controversial figures in 20th-century American letters. Among his unique gifts was the ability to render classical Chinese text into beautiful and moving English verse. These translations, while suffering comparatively little loss of meaning, retain the flavor and sensibility of the original Chinese prose. The New Directions edition includes the Chinese texts of both the *Da Xue* and *Zhong Yong.*

Sues, Ilona Ralf, *Shark's Fin and Millet,* New York: Little Brown and Co., 1944

This is a fascinating look at China that focuses on the conflict between the Guomindang (Nationalist Party) and the Gongchangdang (Chinese Communist Party). Ms. Sues was once a functionary in the WHO anti-opium initiative and found herself in China doing publicity for Jiang Jie Shi (Chiang Kai-shek). For anyone who wants to understand this pivotal period of modern Chinese history, this book offers an inside look at the rigors of political intrigue. It also presents a sympathetic appraisal of the Communist efforts to mobilize the peasantry and defeat the Japanese invaders.

Veith, Ilza (tr.), *Yellow Emperor's Classic of Internal Medicine,* Berkeley: University of California Press, 1972

Ilza Veith's translation of China's oldest extant medical classic has become somewhat of a pillar in the structure of American understanding of Chinese medicine. As a relatively early entry in the field of translation of ancient medical texts, it reflects many of the challenges facing non-Chinese in the study of ancient literary sources.

BOOKS IN CHINESE

Huáng Dì Nèi Jīng Rén Mín Wèi Shēng Chū Bǎn Shè 1986

Nán Jīng (Qīng)

Shāng Hán Lùn (Qīng)

Lēi Jīng Fù Yì (Qīng)

Qiān Jīn Fāng Huá Xià Chū Bǎn Shè 1993

Shuō Wén Jiě Zì Zhōng Huá Shū Jú 1963

Hàn Yǔ Dà Zì Diǎn Sì Chuān Cí Shū Chū Bǎn Shè, Hú Běi Cí Shū Chū Bǎn Shè 1993

Sūn Zǐ Quán Yì Guì Zhōu Rén Mín Chū Bǎn Shè 1992

Chǔ Cí Quán Yì Guì Zhōu Rén Mín Chū Bǎn Shè 1984

Zhuáng Zǐ Quán Yì Guì Zhōu Rén Mín Chū Bǎn Shè 1991

Yì Gǔ Wén Shàng Hái Kē Jì Chū Bǎn Shè 1986

Zhōng Guó Yì Xué Shǐ Hú Nán Kē Xué Jì Shù Chū Bǎn Shè 1985

Xing Mìng Guī Zǐ Běi Jīng Bái Yún Guān

Shuān Méi Yǐng Àn Cóng Shū Hǎi Nán Guó Jì Xīn Wén Chū Bǎn Shè Zhōng Xīn 1995

Index

Imperial Bureau of Rectifying Medical Texts: 115
Imperial Dietician: 53
Inner Canon: 116, 221, 223, 232
integrated medicine: 168
internal elixir: 154, 187, 191, 219

J

jade liquid: 183
Jesuits: 166
jiá gǔ wén: 103
Jiá Yí: 3
jiàn: 44, 210-211
Jiào Zhèng Yī Shū Jú: 148
jiě biǎo: 239-240
Jin Shao: 3
jīn yè: 213-214
jīng: 33, 66-67, 69-70, 72, 84, 104, 132, 152, 154, 172, 174-179, 189-190, 196, 209-210, 212, 215, 218-219, 221, 249
jīng luò: 32-33, 48, 104, 114, 128, 196-197, 217-218, 226, 235, 238, 248
jīng qì: 66, 70, 72, 152, 154, 172, 179, 196, 212, 215, 219, 249
jiǔ zhāng suàn shù: 138
Johnson, Samuel: 200
joy and anger: 49
jǔ àn xún: 230
jūn chén fù zǐ: 57
jūn chén zuǒ shǐ: 96, 238
Jung, Carl: 255

K

Kuhn, Thomas: 137, 168

L

Language of the Pulse: 165
Lao Zi: 2-3, 16, 81-82, 84-86, 121-125, 127, 150, 189, 191, 257-258
Lèi Jīng Fù Yì: 110
Leibniz: 106

lǐ: 14, 95, 105, 220, 224, 226, 243
Li Dong Yuan: 162
Lǐ Jì: 105, 224
lì niào shèn shī: 242
lì qì: 242
Li Shi Zhen: 163
lì xuè: 242
Life and Death: 72-73, 75, 77, 100, 208, 229
Lin Yu Tang: 50, 74, 79-80, 98, 258
líng guāng: 190, 205
Líng Shū: 209-215, 217-218, 220, 222, 234, 237
liù fǔ: 215-216
Liu He Jian: 162
liù qì: 223, 228-229
longevity: 57, 59, 83, 111, 169-173, 175, 177, 179-181, 183-185, 187, 189, 191, 193
Lùn Yǔ: 128
Luo Shu: 110
lycium berries: 52

M

mǎ qián zǐ: 89
Ma Wang Dui: 83, 103, 171
magic: 43, 45, 82, 106, 125, 151, 186-187, 189, 192, 220, 247
mài: 60, 155, 165, 217-220
Mài Jīng: 155
Mài Yǔ: 165
male wū: 44
mankind: 49, 72, 82, 84, 89, 151, 201, 203, 208, 229, 255
Mao Ze Dong: 20, 65, 167
marriage: 54-55, 73, 149
Medicinal Canon of Shen Nong: 96
medicinal formula: 53
meditation: 84, 88-89, 91, 171, 184, 186, 253
Mèng Zǐ: 128
meridians: 32, 48
mǐ: 69

WHO CAN RIDE THE DRAGON?

WHO CAN RIDE THE DRAGON?